A Hallucinogenic Tea, Laced with Controversy

AYAHUASCA IN THE AMAZON AND THE UNITED STATES

Marlene Dobkin de Rios
and Roger Rumrrill

PRAEGER

Westport, Connecticut
London

Library of Congress Cataloging-in-Publication Data

Dobkin de Rios, Marlene.
  A hallucinogenic tea, laced with controversy : ayahuasca in the Amazon and the United States /
  Marlene Dobkin de Rios and Roger Rumrrill.
    p. ; cm.
  Includes bibliographical references and index.
  ISBN 978–0–313–34542–5 (alk. paper)
1. Ayahuasca—Psychotropic effects.   I. Rumrrill, Róger. II. Title.
[DNLM: 1.   Banisteriopsis—South America. 2.   Banisteriopsis—United States. 3.   Hallucinogens—
South America. 4.   Hallucinogens—United States. 5.   Drug and Narcotic Control—history—South
America. 6.   Drug and Narcotic Control—history—United States. 7.   Ethnopharmacology—South
America. 8.   Ethnopharmacology—United States. 9.   Plant Preparations—therapeutic use—South
America. 10.   Plant Preparations—therapeutic use—United States. 11.   Shamanism—history—South
America. 12.   Shamanism—history—United States.   QV 77.7 D633ha 2008]
BF209.A93D63 2008
394.1'4—dc22   2008008793

British Library Cataloguing in Publication Data is available.

Library of Congress Catalog Card Number: 2008008793
ISBN-13: 978–0–313–34542–5

First published in 2008

Praeger Publishers, 88 Post Road West, Westport, CT 06881
An imprint of Greenwood Publishing Group, Inc.
www.praeger.com

Printed in the United States of America

The paper used in this book complies with the
Permanent Paper Standard issued by the National
Information Standards Organization (Z39.48–1984).

10 9 8 7 6 5 4 3 2 1

CONTENTS

CHAPTER 1

INTRODUCTION

A woody vine, brown in color, not particularly interesting to look at, and with no particular odor, winding its way around foliage in the tropical Amazonian rain forests of Peru, Brazil, Ecuador, Bolivia, and Venezuela. A purge, a diuretic, a plant whose stems can be pounded and boiled, and watched for several hours, to produce a foul-tasting drink—a tea called *ayahuasca* in Spanish, or *hoasca* in Portuguese. Why on earth would anyone want to drink this unpleasant brew that causes vomiting and diarrheas for most of those who drink it? Certainly, in the West, such emetic effects are reason to call "911" or to quickly find an urgent care facility to stem the "illness." Yet, in moist tropics of the world, where helminthic disease is widespread, where the spores of intestinal worms are airborne, and where unhygienic conditions abound, a good mother will purge her children periodically. The concept of a purge under those circumstances is a positive experience, one that speaks to compassion and caregiving.

Yet when used as part of healing or spiritual activity, this hallucinogenic plant causes a number of effects on the human organism. The consciousness changes are less than six hours' duration, beginning 30–40 minutes after the individual drinks the potion and reaching a peak after two hours. By six hours, they are pretty much finished. There is cardiovascular stimulation, with moderate increases in heart rate and diastolic blood pressure. The typical psychedelic effects occurring with ayahuasca that have been described for the last 50 years include visual or auditory stimulation, the blending of sensory modalities—synesthesia—and psychological introspection that can include great elation, fear, illumination, or depression. Called "the purge" in Spanish, the drink is often seen to offer spiritual or physical cleansing.

To date there are no real long-term studies of the effects of ayahuasca on human beings. Yet we know that ayahuasca (the term we shall use in this book) has a long history of several thousand years of use, both as a plant medicine and as a spiritual aid, given the psychedelic properties of the vine and its additives. Ayahuasca has been used ritually by diverse groups, ranging from tribal men and women in the heart of the Amazonian rain forest to rural peasants who cultivate rice, beans, and vegetable crops, and who fish in the numerous rivers. Also included in the mix are urban healers with a mixed European and indigenous heritage. People of this ethnicity are called *mestizos* and for the last four centuries have been subject to missionary zeal and converted to Christianity. Urban, middle-class members of new religions with African and European influences have discovered ayahuasca in the last 75 years. Most recently and as a harbinger of the future, ayahuasca has landed on North American shores. Its use has been found allowable by the U.S. Supreme Court when taken within the religious framework of the new Brazilian religion called the União do Vegetal (the UDV), in its American church headquarters in Santa Fe, New Mexico. While legitimate use of ayahuasca as a sacrament is permitted in new religions like the UDV, and others in Brazil, there is also a disturbing development in Europe, the United States, and Canada—we call this phenomenon "drug tourism." It has been around for more than 40 years and has been getting worse each year. Westerners take tours throughout areas of the Amazon and experience "borrowed mysticism." The drink ayahuasca is given to them by new, often false shamans—so-called "technicians of ecstasy"—charlatans who are on the lookout to profit from altering their clients' consciousness. To understand this phenomenon, which is growing in leaps and bounds, netting millions of dollars a year at the expense of those victimized by these Amazonian con men, we also need to look closely at the history of shamanism in the Amazon, as well as at ayahuasca in its many historic manifestations.

With the U.S. Supreme Court decision in February 2006 that permits ayahuasca to be used as a religious sacrament, we see history in the making! The last few years have seen a fierce battle to gain acceptance of the sacramental use of ayahuasca, and it is worth examining so that we can understand the type of arguments offered by the U.S. government opposing the incorporation of ayahuasca into religious ritual. Contrary to this position are the religious beliefs of the União do Vegetal and the contention that ayahuasca heightens spiritual experience through its sacramental effects.

We then turn to an exposé of drug trafficking in shamanic plants to understand how these new developments destroy both native and urban use of traditional ayahuasca healing. Shamanic voices, perspectives of native Amazonian shamans who have legitimate status in their society—as well as new rogue healers—emerge from interviews conducted by the authors, as well as information derived from field anthropologists busy at work in Peru, Venezuela, and Brazil.

Public health issues are of primary concern to us, as new urban shamans frequently dispense powerful chemicals and mixtures of "witchcraft" plants[1] (often in the nightshade family) to their clients. These mixtures are poisonous and interact with foods and medicines. They can cause major illness, disability, and even death. Americans and Europeans are wooed by these pseudo-shamans and their agents or publicists who travel the world to drum up business abroad. The issue of unsupervised and nonmedical use of powerful, mind-altering substances among a naïve and often troubled foreign audience brings to mind European witchcraft with nightshades and daturas, or even a rerun of 1960s American drug use. Several traditional ayahuasca healers with whom we spoke are opposed to the drug tourism that contributes to the demise of their own society's traditions and rituals. And then, there are the postmodern nay-sayers who see history as a set of mere power relationships. They argue that ayahuasca use has always been in flux and that we are simply seeing a new chapter in global change—universal access to the ayahuasca-induced altered state for personal and spiritual needs of visitors from first world European and American societies.

Finally, we integrate themes of drugs, religion, mysticism, and healing within a global context and examine yet another failure of the War on Drugs. There is little attempt made to stem the exploitation of individuals who are given powerful plant hallucinogens in a jungle setting. Certainly, anthropologists must take responsibility for their own role in promoting hallucinogenic use in a global perspective, even from their scholarly perch. Ayahuasca information has permeated this internet highway on which we surf and has diffused down to the global marketplace.[2] At last count, "ayahuasca tours" brought more than 45,100 hits on search engines and "ayahuasca" alone brought 908,000, as Western men and women are eager to learn about new ways to experience drug-induced altered states.

In the last chapter, we examine the future of ayahuasca—in healing, and sacramentally, within a religious setting. The U.S. Supreme Court decision in February 2006 is quite unique and suggests that other religious challenges for sacramental use of psychedelics in the years to come may be successful as well.

A Word About the Authors

Both of us have dedicated many years to the study of the Amazon. Marlene de Rios lived in Iquitos, Peru for a year during 1968–1969 while gathering data on ayahuasca healers for her doctoral dissertation at the University of California–Riverside. She returned to the Amazon on sabbatical leave from teaching anthropology at California State University–Fullerton in 1977 and worked intensively with don Hilde, a mestizo healer in Pucallpa, Peru, and his clientele. Then, from 1997 to 2005, she worked with the União do Vegetal Church in Brazil and visited four Brazilian cities, including Manaus, and eleven UDV temples, in order to better understand the role of ayahuasca as a sacrament in their church.

Roger Rumrrill, a writer, was born in Iquitos in the Peruvian Amazon and worked for many years as a journalist, being interested in ecological and political issues. He is past director of the Center for Indigenous Cultures of Peru (CHIRAPAQ) and is an internationally recognized authority on the Amazon jungle, to which he travels on a regular basis. At present, he is a consultant to indigenous organizations in the Amazon basin area as well as a Peruvian congressional advisor on drugs and the Amazon region.

Our joint interests enable us to have a clear vision of the Amazon and of the place of ayahuasca, both in the world we live in and in the years to come.

CHAPTER 2

NATIVE USE OF AYAHUASCA

In this chapter we will look at the use of ayahuasca by native peoples of South America, as well as at traditional *mestizo* healers working within a long-standing tradition of healing. We will also look at social and cultural changes in the Peruvian Amazon and how they have affected ayahuasca use today, particularly in the form of drug tourism. Then we will turn in Chapter 4 to take a detailed look at the neo-shamans, or new healers—some good, some bad, some horrendous—as well as at the dangers of this drug tourism.

The area of native ayahuasca use extends from the northern area of Colombia to eastern Bolivia in the south, to Venezuela and Guyana in the north. The eastern extension has gone as far as Paria, Brazil, at the mouth of the Amazon. In addition to its visionary powers, the plant has a reputation for bestowing paranormal power on the user, supposedly to allow the user to read the minds of others or to recognize negative emotions used to harm individuals and communities. Anthropological literature suggests that the plant also stimulates mental abilities and enables people to suppress hunger. De Rios long ago pointed out the anxiety-reducing properties of the tea. The Australian anthropologist Robin Rodd[1] believes that the use of this plant by indigenous peoples can contribute to harmonizing the emotions of groups and in this way, it promotes social stability. During intoxication with ayahuasca, the Piaroa native peoples of southern Venezuela, studied by Rodd,[2] engage in sorcery battles to rid themselves of the bewitchment they believe to be sent to them by malevolent shamans. These people believe that such powerful individuals can even kill people and can cause long-term suffering to communities. When negative emotions prevent people from working and relating to one another, a shaman is called in to deflect these negative emotions away from the victims by sorcery attack. Visions induced by ayahuasca potions and a psychedelic snuff, *yopo,* are used to help the shaman understand the nature of the social relations and to return the evil to the malevolent sender.

Siskind in 1973[3] showed how in-marrying husbands in Amazonian indigenous groups, strangers to one another, would take ayahuasca to be of one heart, to work well together, and to share the fruits of their labor. Shamans in the moist South American tropics who work with ayahuasca have used the plant to heal as well as to bewitch enemies. The shamans are believed to communicate with spirit helpers, or familiars, and to be able either to cause entry of a dart (*virote*) into the body of an enemy or to extract pathogenic agents introduced into a client's body by an enemy shaman. The visions that accompany the tea help the shamans do battle with enemies from other tribes, as well as to predict the future. Shamans gain insight into practical problems to help them to make day-to-day decisions. Ayahuasca can also enhance empathy to help shamans perceive the motivations and desires of others, their feelings, and their states of mind. The successful shaman can bring about social harmony by allowing individuals to profoundly understand others with whom they work—mind you, we are talking about tribal societies where leaders can lead, but followers do not have to follow if they are not so inclined. Ayahuasca aids the shaman in resonating psychologically with his neighbors.

Early reports in the Amazon rain forest cite how ayahuasca was taken to give the hunter strength and the ability to avoid malevolent spirits. Night vision, too, is said to be enhanced by drinking the tea. Like other psychedelics and substances that suppress hunger, ayahuasca can be very important in making it so that rations do not have to be brought along on the hunt. The stimulant property of ayahuasca may increase work output,[4] along with causing powerful visions. High dosages of ayahuasca stimulate the visual cortex and also bring about increased empathy among users. The neurobiologist Riba[5] found that the effects of ayahuasca influenced attention, emotion, and memory—an area only recently being studied scientifically. Modification of the way people think about life, in general, is also part and parcel of the ayahuasca experience. Any substance that sharpens interpersonal awareness and increases empathy, especially in a group setting, can produce social bonding and bring participants closer together.

The history of ayahuasca use in the Amazon is interesting to examine. Even today in the Amazonian tropical rain forest, over 50,000 indigenous peoples who are nomadic hunters and gatherers still practice incipient agriculture. They were never conquered by their Incan neighbors to the west. There was commerce and trade, at least to a limited degree, between the rain forest and the highlands and perhaps even coastal areas. We see, for example, many similarities between the ayahuasca use within rain forest tribes described by anthropologists and contemporary mescaline healing in the coastal areas. Without doubt, herbal medicines and healing techniques moved from one region to another in pre-Colombian times. Once the Spanish established control in the sixteenth century, native Indian medical lore blended with Andalusian Spanish folk beliefs about illness and its treatment. Cartomancy from Italy and Spain became integrated into these techniques, which spread from the European soldiers of fortune to the emerging mestizo peasants in the Spanish colonies.

Native medicine among Peruvian Indians at the time of the conquest, for example, was probably as effective as that which prevailed among the Spaniards. Since there were few physicians during this period, the Spanish soldiers highly regarded medical practice in Indian towns, and many Indian medicinal plants and herbs were used by missionaries. We will see later on the effectiveness of plants like ayahuasca and of secondary tobacco smoke to provide antianxiety and antidepressive effects.

The drug tourism to be discussed in Chapter 5 is not the first time that quackery and dishonesty in the practice of medicine and dispensing of drugs has occurred. As early as 1535, the Spanish throne was issuing royal decrees against con men stiffing the public. Over the centuries a rich pharmacopoeia of plant drugs and medicines found their way into the general home remedies of the region. The contemporary native peoples continue to live in communities difficult to access, along major river systems. Their way of life has been markedly changed by the encroachment of civilization. The shamanic healing traditions have become altered in form but nonetheless are still very much alive. Many of these native Americans have become "mestizoized" and have emerged as rural farmers near cities like Iquitos and Pucallpa. Influences of Roman Catholic proselytization, mixed with medieval metaphysical beliefs, and influenced by evangelical Protestantism, are widespread.

However, dangers abound in taking ayahuasca. While the general scientific overview of indole hallucinogens is that they are generally safe when drunk in their traditional formulations prepared by seasoned healers, nonetheless new data are emerging which provoke some real concerns about ayahuasca's use. This is especially so when the tea is administered by individuals who are untrained and who simply want to make a quick buck, not being particularly attentive to any potential dangers. For example, de Rios[6] reported that an epileptic informant in Iquitos was given ayahuasca, and during a seizure that followed, she fell into the river and drowned.

Ayahuasca has the ability to raise blood pressure, although hypertensive crises have not been widely reported. There are, however, food interactions which can cause problems for those drinking the tea. There is a class of chemicals called beta-carbolines in ayahuasca that have the potential to interact dangerously with other drugs such as amphetamines and MDMA (ecstasy), as well as antidepressive and antianxiety medicines like Prozac, Paxil, Zoloft, Luvox, Celexa, Lexapro, and Effexor, to name a few. Moreover, certain foods that are commonplace in Western diets can cause additional problematic drug interactions. Foods that are fermented or processed are among those presenting problems and include your average bologna sandwich, or any other smoked or cured meats. Protein extracts, soy foods, and even the pod of the fava bean (said to have a large quantity of the neurochemical dopamine) can cause adverse reactions. Protein foods and beverages at room temperature need to be avoided as well. Also on the list of dietary restrictions are foods containing a high amount of tyramine; fermented or processed foods with bacteria and fungi, such as aged cheese; liver products; and concentrated yeast. Additionally, foods such as sauerkraut, red meat, tap beer, and some wines, such as Chianti, can be problematic. In the past, traditional ayahuasca diets were bland before the individual took ayahuasca—free from salt, spices, sugar, and fats. Moreover, men were cautioned not to have sex prior to the experience (perhaps there would be some changes in testosterone levels that could diminish the ayahuasca experience). Such a diet, along with fasting before the session, increased brain serotonin, minimizing vomiting and diarrheas. Traditional healers historically have been very fussy about the diets they set up for their clients' ingestion before and after ayahuasca use. Diets often included chicken, fish, plantains, seeds, nuts, and starches.

One fatal intoxication[7] has been reported in a scientific journal—probably a suicide, as the autopsy showed a number of drugs in high concentrations added to a homemade ayahuasca brew. Another case whispered about among Iquitos residents concerned a woman who died from an aneurysm while under the effects of ayahuasca. Since she had this preexisting condition, her family did not press charges against the ayahuasca healer.

Aboriginal Use of Ayahuasca

Ayahuasca has many names in native American languages, including *natema* and *caapi*—along with the Portuguese term, hoasca. It has been part of Amazonian culture perhaps as long as 8,000 years and has allowed native peoples to communicate with spirits of the dead and spirits of the earth. Prophecy is one of the main motivations that native peoples had to seek out ayahuasca intoxication. The tea is drunk in darkness since it is perceived to be more powerful that way and is believed to enhance healing. To make the tea, one boils the ayahuasca vine for several hours in a covered pot with 24 ounces of water. The contents slowly boil away, leaving a thick, viscous syrup behind.

Historically, ayahuasca was believed to provoke telepathic properties in the user, which allowed Indians to describe faraway houses, castles, and cities that had white people moving about in them. The chemical properties of the plant contain harmine, an alkaloid synthesized from Syrian rue (*Peganum harmala*). The seeds of this plant were used in the Middle East and were probably known to the ancient Greeks. In Italy and Spain, the seeds of Syrian rue were used as a vermifuge and diuretic. Even in the early years of the twentieth century, a second plant which natives added to the brew in its preparation was described by Reko.[8] Called *chacruna* in Spanish, the plant (*Psychotropia viridis*) contains dimethyltryptamine (DMT), a powerful psychedelic listed as a Schedule I substance in the United States. The addition of *Psychotropia viridis* greatly heightens the visual effects of the tea.

Shamanism in the Old Days

Ayahuasca has played an important role in the past, in the techniques of the hunt, among indigenous peoples. These Amazon hunters, called *mitayeros,* took great care in their diets and purged themselves with ayahuasca to cleanse themselves from bad luck, called "saladera" in Spanish. After taking ayahuasca, the hunters would bathe with leaves, roots, and medicinal plant cuttings, which were supposed to change the odor of the human body, very strong and characteristic, easily perceived by the forest animals. The plant baths were to change human odors to resemble the forest, to confuse the animals and their powerful olfactory senses. The hunter could then follow the path of the deer, a very clever and intelligent creature, without being detected. The deer and other animals could detect the odor of a hunter without this preparation at more than 100 meters' distance, as the strong human odor came in front of him. It is possible that these habits went back many thousands of years, enabling the hunters to trap the "spirit" of the animal facilitating the hunt, owed mainly to the use of ayahuasca.

The indigenous and mestizo Amazonic hunters also trained and prepared their dogs to specialize in a certain type of hunt. These animals were treated in the same way that human hunters were, but the mouth of the animal was also cleaned and rinsed with a combination of medicinal leaves. The animal refined its olfaction to smell the prey at far away distances. The dog would be submitted to a rigorous diet. He would be kept hungry for several days and then made to smell the skin of the deer or whichever animal of the forest the dog was to specialize in hunting. Different dogs would be trained to aid in the hunt of a particular animal in this manner.

Hallucinogens and Addiction

Overall, hallucinogens like ayahuasca have one of the lowest potentials of developing dependence among individuals. Perhaps five percent of those who ingest teas made from the ayahuasca vine mixed with the chacruna leaf would meet psychiatric diagnostic criteria for drug dependence. Moreover, no chronic diseases or medical conditions are associated with hallucinogens like ayahuasca, and we may find in the future that these substances might even be useful in the treatment of neurological disorders like Parkinson's disease. The primary concern of the scholar and of public health officials is what happens when an individual with some underlying psychological disorder, such as severe depression, anxiety, or schizophrenia, drinks the tea—even if in a ritual setting, and even when accompanied by a skilled guide. Enduring psychoses can still develop under these circumstances.[9] Additionally, individuals' judgments are sometimes impaired during hallucinogenic use and thus they might suffer injury. There are particularly adverse effects in perception and emotion, with one of the most problematic effects being that of panic, psychotic-like confusion, and disorientation—still more reason why these substances need to be used in a controlled setting, either medical or religious, with a skilled guide present to respond to and minimize any of these problems.

In an early study by Dr. Oscar Janiger,[10] from 1954–1962, on LSD effects among almost 1,000 men and women in Los Angeles, California, results showed overwhelming, initially negative themes among the research subjects. Themes such as fear, anxiety, panic, and so forth, were found among these naïve users who were given pure Sandoz LSD long before any literature existed to set up expectations for particular visionary experiences. In this context, ayahuasca has hardly been a household name among those who find their way to the Amazon, until recent years. Most have had rather vague expectations of how the tea will alter their normal waking consciousness.

Ayahuasca and Tobacco Use

We cannot really talk about ayahuasca without looking at the accompanying tobacco use. We know that ayahuasca has properties that reduce anxiety. Now, we look at *Tabaco rustica,* a wild species of tobacco, which has been widely used throughout Amazonian history for its prophylactic powers to heal, according to native lore. De Rios would often return to her home in Iquitos in 1968–1969 after observing an ayahuasca session and reek from tobacco smoke which the healer had blown over her head and neck area. This is said to keep *mal aires* (evil vapors) in the street from harming an individual. Much to the authors' surprise, recent studies by researchers at the University of California–Irvine throw some light on this shamanic behavior.

A recent publication looks at smoking by adolescents to self-medicate attentional and emotional dysfunctions. While the focus of the research is youth who suffer specific psychiatric syndromes and who are susceptible to smoking in excess of the expected level in a control group, the data are very suggestive.[11] Findings show that nicotine and other constituents of tobacco have a significant effect on neural circuitry that underlies the regulation of attention and affect. Even secondary smoke is involved—in our case, smoke that is blown over the patient and blown into the ayahuasca potion to be imbibed. This use resonates back to diminishing depressive and anxiety symptoms. While American youth with attention deficit disorders may smoke tobacco to self-medicate themselves, it would appear that South American shamans who widely use tobacco in their rituals are also using the secondary smoke to diminish the negative emotions of their clients. Nicotine is known to have anxiety-reducing properties. Most of the clients benefit from this secondary smoke, both traditionally among river-edge peasants and peasants in cities, as well in recent decades among foreigners seeking ayahuasca healing. The shamanic healer uses tobacco as his ally. While he may be totally in the dark about the neurochemical reactions of his clients, pragmatic trial and error over millennia have contributed to his knowledge as a healer.

Shamanic Power and Hallucinogens

When we think about hallucinogenic drugs such as ayahuasca, political variables do not generally come to mind. Yet anthropologists have found that in societies of the world existing prior to European contact, when plant hallucinogens were used to achieve non-ordinary states of consciousness for religious or healing purposes, politics often motivated such drug use. As societies became more complex over millennia, access to these plant hallucinogens was controlled and regulated by powerful elite groups. As societies underwent social change and were conquered by others, their drug rituals and esoteric knowledge often were lost to posterity. Clues to these beliefs and rituals, however, remained coded in the art of these cultures.

Among hunters and gatherers, shamans functioned to provide spiritual guidance. In non-nation-states, they were able to exercise control over their peers—such control and domination by shamans was common in these hunting and gathering communities. Access to altered states of consciousness (ASCs) induced by plant hallucinogens provided power to individuals in all levels of society. The shaman guided the hallucinogenic experience and created exceptional emotional states among his fellows. He was acknowledged by all to have power and dominion over animal and plant familiars, which he could summon at will to do his bidding. These plant hallucinogens were used to achieve contact with the spiritual realms and to allow the shaman to magically manipulate supernatural forces for social purposes. In a loosely structured society, the shaman could define and control good and evil, manipulate and express power relationships, and exercise magical control over nature.

Power is a topic that has challenged anthropologists for many decades. In tribal societies, the source of power to bewitch and to cause illness or misfortunes to others has historically been seen as residing outside of the self. In the Amazon region studied by de Rios,[12] ayahuasca played an important role in this world view where evil men and women would be able to bewitch their enemies and cause them illness, bad luck, and even death. Utilizing the visionary property of the plants, the first step in this drama was for the mestizo shaman to identify the suspected evildoer. He did this by calling upon his animal or plant familiars, who instructed him in understanding the etiology of the illness or bewitchment. Then, he would return the evil to its perpetrator; in the process, the man or woman seeking help could be treated with plant medicines. What a difference from the psychodynamic world view of Freud and contemporary Western psychology. In the latter case, the etiology of psychological disorders and stress are clearly anchored within the individual's self (although influenced by his milieu), but they are not attributed to evil-willing on the part of one's enemies or rivals. Nor is illness in Western societies believed to be caused by powerful spirit forces. In shamanic- and mestizo-based societies, one can argue that power strengthens the individual. When forces outside the individual govern what a person does to such an extent that the individual is no longer in control of him- or herself, people then become dependent because they can feel strong only when they are near a source of strength. Is it possible that the need to rely on a powerful ayahuasca healer to guide one's hallucinogenic journey is the concept that motivates the drug tourists who visit the Amazon? We will look at this in Chapter 3. Certainly the journey is long and arduous, as tourists ingest a foul-smelling, foul-tasting substance to obtain insightful visions that are carefully interpreted by powerful shamanic guides. Perhaps "power" may mean that the neo-shaman is able to cash in on good fortune—perhaps charge outrageous prices for his services, buy property, develop botanical gardens, and travel abroad? The neo-shaman can use the power of ayahuasca to persuade, to bargain with, and to manipulate others.

Another manifestation of power deals with the concept of duty and honor. A traditional shaman such as don Hilde,[13] discussed in this chapter, sees himself as an instrument of a higher authority (in don Hilde's case, Christ). His personal goals are subordinated to this higher authority. With Amazonian modernization and urbanization, we are not as frequently seeing shamans using their powers as a service directed toward the well-being of the community. In the past, the traditional mestizo healers appear to have had a higher moral and ethical approach compared to the new shamans who typically seduce and then cast aside female followers or who exhibit crass financial motives. During the long years of don Hilde's work in healing, he accepted donations and never turned people away simply because they had no money to pay him.

If we look at political power from the anthropologist's perspective, we can characterize human prehistory into four major types of societies, which range from egalitarian hunter and gatherer societies to ranked horticultural societies, to intensive agricultural societies that are stratified, to finally the state-level societies. In egalitarian societies having shamanism as the religious system, the shaman evokes his authority, although he does not have access to coercion, nor is he able to impose any sanctions—the behavior of others is not a response to threat or the use of punishment. In these hunting and gathering societies, an individual wields power simply by means of personal strength, influence, and authority. There are no orders of dominance or paramountcy. In egalitarian societies like those found historically in the Amazon, one individual generally is not able to tell people to behave in a certain way. In ranked societies with an economic basis of horticulture and hunting, we find that leaders can lead, but followers may decide not to follow. Often leaders have to set a good example so that peers will mimic their behavior. As social stratification emerges over time, more people come to exert power. In state-level societies, warfare and killing become monopolies of the state and are carried out only at certain times, in certain places, and under the specific conditions set by the state in a legal manner, with the state having armies, militia, or police forces to maintain social order.

For some scholars, the central idea of shamanistic religion is the establishment by humans of contact with the supernatural world. This is done by entering into a trance state with the help of an intermediary, a shaman. Primary to this religious system is belief in an accessible supernatural world and the ability of humans to contact and even control it. The shaman is an agent who works on behalf of a group, although generally with an individual and not a congregation. The shaman is inspired by helping spirits, called familiars, generally of the animal kingdom, as well as being inspired by the extraordinary ecstatic experience he or she has.

Our concern with current neo-shamanism is that the exercise of power often consists of these new shamans exhibiting a megalomaniacal style in the presence of followers who are intoxicated by powerful hallucinogens that open them up to suggestion. At the least, this practice offends our sense of fairness and also the need to guarantee public safety. In tribal societies of antiquity, the shamans (and there were numerous individuals in this role) were spiritual guardians of the community. They were believed to control forces that were more powerful than the individual or more powerful than society could control on its own. The individual and the group gained ontological security through the fact that these ways of accumulating and exercising power would have been adaptive, given the low level of control that the society's members possessed over resources. Shamans were obliged to confront and combat their groups' adversaries, heal diseases, and neutralize misfortunes caused by enemies. They were believed able to obtain magical powers and to transform themselves into powerful animal figures which they used to rectify evil or to redress harm. They descended to nether worlds to consult with ancestral spirits and traveled to celestial realms where they returned with special information and predictions of future events. Plant hallucinogens were the glue that enabled a shaman to obtain and demonstrate his powers. In European and American societies today we find a real prevalence of romanticization of the role of the shaman. Elements of these ancient and pervasive belief systems have persisted over the centuries and are ubiquitous. Nowadays in the United States or Europe, one can easily pay for weekend training to have an out-of-body experience or to learn to introspect or to acquire a power familiar by drumming or through breathing exercises. Men and women today exercise very little control over their physical and psychological environments. The need to dominate their milieux, however tenuously, can be ameliorated by taking hallucinogens in an exotic setting with a presumed powerful guide. The exceptional emotional states evoked by the shamanic healer depend on his acts of dominion and posturing. In traditional societies individuals may believe that power resides in the hallucinogenic plants provided by powerful omnipotent individuals. They then cure individuals, route their enemies and provide ontological security. Even Skinner[14] wrote, "human beings do not have the freedom to choose what they think they have, and that their behavior is controlled by forces in the environment outside of themselves. Because of this, it is essential that they acknowledge superior strength and power of the contingencies that control their behavior."

Suggestibility and Hallucinogens

A relatively little-discussed aspect of plant hallucinogens like ayahuasca is the way that the biochemical properties of the plants can evoke suggestibility within those who ingest them. We do know that this ability to influence consciousness is a psychological characteristic of drug-induced states, as well as being a normal human psychological phenomenon. We could actually call it a "psycho-technology"[15] and document its use cross-culturally to manage youthful ASCs, in order to ensure conformity and adherence to group norms. This practice was done to aid in the survival of the social group, as elders assumed a major role in managing and regulating the hallucinogenic experiences of adolescents in order to create optimally constructive outcomes.

Anthropologists rarely use the term "suggestibility," although the psychological, psychiatric, and hypnosis literature is full of such references, with this word indicating a person's propensity to respond to suggested communications.[16] Or, it can be used to describe a particular state of mind that favors suggestion. The psychologist Eysenck[17] defined suggestion as "a process where one or more persons cause one or more individuals to change without a critical response of their judgments, opinions, attitudes or patterns of behavior." Psychologists are interested in who elicits suggestion, and whether the suggestion is verbal or nonverbal. Is it a request or a command? Is the communicator a high-status individual? When there are moderate levels of anxiety, social influence increases. We know that human consciousness is not a singular and continuous state but a layered system of cognitive control. Information goes along multiple independent pathways. Willpower, self-initiative, and critical awareness provide an individual with higher levels of control. But a person can disengage from that control under different circumstances.[18]

If we observe shamanic activity taking place through dance, movement, repetitive ritual, or drug ingestion, we can see that many of these practices fall into the area of dissociative behavior. The individual no longer is involved in higher-order executive control functions. The individual's conscious monitoring authority is overridden in the dissociative state.

Biologically speaking, suggestibility can be seen as a device that gives the individual a way to adapt to harsh reality—by means of denial, illusion, and false or overly optimistic beliefs. This enables the person to cope with stress and conflicts in his environment and confers crucial survival advantage. Human beings appear to have evolved as suggestible animals because of survival needs. Suggestibility allows an individual to transcend reality, become cohesive with his social group, allow himself to discharge negative emotions, and turn away from himself—a good escape from trauma and irreconcilable conflict. The psychological concept of "bounded rationality"[19] is useful here, defined as the human tendency to learn from others or to accept social influence. Individuals who are quick to act without weighing all the probabilities may have, in fact, enhanced their survivability. At the same time, individuals who are docile, who accept suggestions without independent evaluation of the circumstances, can achieve an extra ability to survive in hostile environments. This suggestibility is marked by the presence of hundreds of thousands of different religions that span human history. Information is beginning to be synthesized that suggests that hallucinogenic drugs enhance primary suggestibility to a degree comparable to that produced by hypnosis itself.

Psychedelic substances like ayahuasca create a state of hypersuggestiblity in which persons are very open to being influenced by others.[20] Many traditional cultures have utilized this condition to inculcate cultural values and behaviors in young people as they receive initiation into adulthood. In the West, countercultural values can be inculcated in young people when using these psychedelics, especially when using them in an antinomian context. Grob and de Rios have written about tribal societies where psychedelics were used to create a bonding experience among young men who were obliged to cooperate in the food quest, or among young women undergoing a short-term educational experience prior to marrying and bearing children. In these tribal settings, expectations of youth prior to their first experience with the substance were major, and the beliefs and practices allowed them a culturally recognized framework within which to anticipate and interpret the experience they would have. A true psychedelic sacrament would be one, as Baker has written,[21] with "religiously justified rituals that establish and promote a person's identity within the group and affirm the core values of a society." Such is hardly the case with the drug tourists, but more like to be so with the União do Vegetal Church (UDV) members.

What has not received enough attention, in our opinion, is the major role of these plants in fostering suggestibility. Call it mind control, if you like, or brainwashing—but suggestibility is the more accurate psychological term in current use. Some interesting scientific literature exists that links plants like ayahuasca both to the impairment of memory (both storage and retrieval) and to submissive and obedient behavior in victims who are given psychedelics as a type of "Mickey Finn." In such states, the intoxicated individual follows any command, presents no resistance, and offers money and possessions to the offender. Brief information processing can be impaired with some of the psychedelics. Moreover, individuals have increased susceptibility of accepting or responding to specific statements when hallucinogens are ingested, such as agreeing that they see a particular deity. This submissive behavior is probably the result of hallucinogens that normally control emotional behavior, particularly aggressive behavior, acting on the brain structures. The daturas may have an inhibitory action on the limbic system—on the hippocampus and amygdala, which control aggression and learning and the display of defense responses. Cognitive functioning, psychomotor facility and coordination, and expression of emotion were perceived to be very similar to trance states produced by hypnosis, intense reverie, sleep deprivation, and similar interventions. Hallucinogenic drugs such as ayahuasca may enhance primary suggestibility to a degree comparable to that produced by inducing hypnosis. Subjects experiencing hallucinogenic states describe intense feelings of detachment or dissociation from the immediate environment and from the self, deep absorption, and feelings that actions and movements were being carried out as though the subject were asleep and as though compelled by a mysterious force. An individual's normal control of voluntary activity coupled with a lack of desire to take the initiative in controlling one's own planning functions can presumably lead to a loss of initiative that increases amenability to the suggestions delivered by an outside source. This phenomenon was described in *Brave New World* by Huxley and was a futuristic vision of a totalitarian society where the world was controlled chemically, and the population was coerced into loving its servitude.

Shamanism and Ontology

A major theme encountered among shamans in hunting and gathering societies of the world is that of shamanic control over nature—animals, plants, and celestial spirits. In tribal societies we find harsh and difficult environments facing human beings who have little predictability over their food resources, given their low-level agricultural and harvesting potentials. Nonetheless, by means of altered states of consciousness induced by plant hallucinogens, individuals believe they can contact nether realms to make spirit forces of plants or animals act on their behalf. Such control makes individuals in these societies feel more secure and satisfied.

This sense of security and optimism about the future appear paradoxical in light of recent archaeological data documenting famine and throughout human prehistory. Certainly global environmental changes during the immediate post-Pleistocene period meant that populations of hunters and gatherers began to grow beyond the carrying capacity of their environment, forcing them to exploit marginal eco-niches.

What psychological characteristics make for a healthy individual? The so-called "biology of hope" is a concept that has gained interest in recent years as applied to the efficacy of folk or shamanic healers. If an individual enters into states of desperation and despair, his immune system is compromised, and disease may occur. Helpless, hopeless men and women overly stressed by their environments can easily develop clinical depression. Psychiatrically, this results in a loss of interest or pleasure in all activities, a lack of reactivity to usually pleasurable stimuli. One's moods do not improve even temporarily should something good happen. Shamanic healers reverse their clients' negative emotions by neutralizing the helplessness and hopelessness that these people experience. This brings to mind the old adage that "nature cures the illness, while the doctor amuses the patient!"[22]

Research in cognitive psychology shows that feelings of pessimism result from strong emotional states. We can assume the same mechanisms were at work in earlier periods of human prehistory. Rather than focusing on depression and the disinclination of a person to respond actively to life's challenges, shamanism is just the opposite. In the belief system of shamanism emphasis is placed on the individual shaman, who can exercise power and control over nature. Members of his group have a secure expectation that sufficient food and water and the fertility of animals and human beings will endure. This "psycho-technology" is significant in enabling groups of people to be successful in the struggle to survive, despite a difficult and often hostile environment. This is a corruption of reality, as hunters and gatherers create illusions of environmental control in order to insulate themselves from the experience of emotional depression. This is necessary, given that fear of imminent starvation or death could cause real trauma to a person's emotional integrity. People create many illusions, and throughout history, illusion and self-deception have existed.

The psychologist Seligman has written about control or power in human society. He has said that if an individual believes that control rests with himself, then that individual holds the certainty that he can do something about a given event. Adverse events appear more predictable. Even shamans who are defeated in a task claim that the victory is due to the superior power of the malevolent spirits of his opponent. Individuals experience less anxiety and arousal when they believe they have some internal power to control events around them.

At some level we can argue that all human beings, whether hunters and gatherers or urban residents in contemporary society, are obsessed with an attempt to dominate the world in which they live. Each person desires to shape his life-world based on his immediate experience. In the shamanic trance state—which Westerners call dissociation—the human brain has the capacity to dissociate itself from its own data and perceive its environment selectively, especially in the way that it processes information and stores and retrieves memories. Anthropologists interested in dissociative states cross-culturally see dissociation as streams of mental activity that are multiple and simultaneous, streams that influence experience. When the individual enters into a dissociated state, he experiences a loss of usual interrelationships between various groups of mental processes, and it is as if there is an independent functioning of each aspect of mental process—each process separated from the rest. Information becomes compartmentalized.

In shamanic states, we see self-deception at work, especially with regard to the illusion that the individual can control his environment. Illusions keep people from experiencing emotional depression. It is as if we are obliged to distort our way of thinking about the control we have over life events. If we fail to do this, depression inevitably follows. Religion—particularly shamanism—evolved to help human beings survive and to enhance their ability to cope.

Spiritist Doctrine in Latin America

In the Brazilian and Peruvian Amazon, ayahuasca has been used by indigenous cultures for thousands of years. Since the late fifteenth century, the use of ayahuasca for religious and healing purposes has occurred among mestizo farmers, generally in locations remote from urban areas. It was derived from shamanic knowledge about the use of these cultigens. Typically, cultural specialists called *ayahuasqueros* controlled these activities. In Brazil, the best-known area of mestizo ayahuasca use was in Acre in the southwest Amazonia, between the Bolivian and Peruvian frontiers. In the populated area of Rio Branco, the capital of Acre, ayahuasca use was very much influenced by a series of religious ideologies. These included Christianity and particularly focused on spiritist and spiritualist schools of esoterism and Kardecism.[23] These schools had roots in European esoteric thought of the nineteenth century. Kardecism emphasized the primacy of the spiritual over the material. Allan Kardec was the nom de plume of Leon Rivail (1804–1869), who published many books and articles that were translated into Spanish and Portuguese and widely distributed throughout Latin America. His focus was to demonstrate the existence and immortality of the soul. He used the term "spiritism," which he saw as denoting a religion, a philosophy, and a science compatible with all religions.

Kardec, from 1854 onward, envisaged his task as being to unify diverse spiritist beliefs. As the result of his effort, there was a resurgence of a real spiritist religion, which gained more and more adepts. His key work,

The Book of the Spirits, according to Kardec was dictated by invisible spirits. It has been translated into many languages and is considered the Bible of the spiritist faith.

Kardec created a moral doctrine that gathered together the romantic and spiritual tendencies of his age. He asserted that it was possible to establish communication with the world of the spirits, in order to console the afflicted and to reveal to them a more transcendent sense of life after death. His movement opened the door to metaphysics for Westerners, and its history is intricately tied up with ayahuasca use among certain groups of traditional mestizo healers, as well as with the two major religions in Brazil that utilize ayahuasca—namely the Santo Daime Church and the União do Vegetal Church.

Kardec's doctrines filtered down to the urban lower classes and peasantry of Latin America and mixed with Brazilian religions like the União do Vegetal, where the founder, Mestre Gabriel, used the term "high spiritism." In fact, the actual name of the UDV defines it as a Christian spiritist religion; it is referred to by adherents with the formal name *Centro Espirita Beneficente União Do Vegetal.* By entering into unusual mental states such as trance, a medium would be able to communicate with spiritual entities on behalf of his clients. This is similar to the belief in the shaman's omnipotent powers to discern such spirit forces and to then dominate and control them for his own needs and purposes. The nineteenth century was a time in which spiritualism reached its heyday, with spirit communications, materializations, and table-knocking widely reported in the press and popular books. By 1850, spiritualism (often used interchangeably with "spiritism" despite differences to be discussed shortly) had spread through the United States, England, Europe, and Latin America, and it was reported in Guatemala and Cuba in the 1850s. By 1865, spiritualism was found in Caracas, Venezuela among high government officials who claimed to have contact with spirits of the highest order.

Kardec was the major intellectual influence on Latin American spiritualism. He believed that the term "spiritualist" meant anyone who believes that a realm exists that contains more than matter. He was interested in demonstrating the existence and immortality of the soul and used the term spiritism rather than spiritualism. He believed that the spiritualists dealt only with occult phenomena, while the beliefs of spiritism were that of a religion, a philosophy, and a science. Kardec was strongly influenced by Hinduism and believed in the concepts of reincarnation and karma, stating that nothing in life is fortuitous, and we cannot escape from the consequences of our acts.

Another intellectual influence was that of Swedenborg, a Swedish mystic who lived from 1688–1772. He was an engineer and metallurgist by profession and wrote 32 books on the world of the spirit. His concept of man's life depending on his relationship with a hierarchy of spirits was influential throughout Latin American spiritist groups. All of life was seen by him to correspond to a hierarchy of beings that represent different orders and yet act in correspondence with each other. There are different levels above and below man, and the spirits affect man's behavior. Like other mystics, Swedenborg recognized that breathing exercises and introspective concentration were essential to realizing mystical unity experiences. His writing including information about both "high" and "low" spirits. The lower spirits seek to possess and control some part of a person's body. The higher-order spirits are rarer and do not oppose the person's will but are helpful guides. Swedenborg conceptualized them as angels who assist a person. Many of these spirits reside in the interior mind, and good spirits have some control over the evil ones. Doctrines, both of Kardec and Swedenborg, became synthesized with beliefs of Afro-Brazilian cults and folk Catholicism in Brazil.

The conditions laid down by Allan Kardec explain the spiritist doctrine as follows:

1. communication with the world of spirits is possible through the phenomenon of mediumship;
2. the soul survives (similar to Christian dogma);
3. the pleasures of the senses are to be deprecated;
4. renunciation and charity are important virtues;
5. reincarnation exists;
6. the existence of the devil and of hell is negated;
7. man is affirmed to possess three parts: a material body that perishes with death; a fluid body or a spiritual wrapping that separates from the body during sleep, hypnosis, and trance, when paranormal manifestations originate; and a perfectible and imperishable spirit.

These beliefs spread from the doctrine's origin in the United States, first to Europe and then Latin America. In the nineteenth century, cultural and commercial exchanges in Latin America were more intense with Europe than with the United States. Many Latin Americans from the middle classes were educated in Europe, thus Kardec's direct influence in Paris made a great impression on esoteric thought, gaining a large number of followers in Brazil, Mexico, and Argentina. In Peru, the doctrine's main route of diffusion was the Amazon. In Iquitos, there was a wave of spiritist practices that resulted in the establishing of many centers in those early years.

Kardec's influence significantly shifted ayahuasca use from small-scale, individually organized sessions of mestizos in Peru and Bolivia to more institutional organizations of ayahuasca-using groups, such as the União do Vegetal and Santo Daime churches. Central Brazil as well has been influenced by the so-called "New Age Movement," in rural and urban zones alike, where ayahuasca is used both within religious and nonreligious formats. This "new religious consciousness" includes ayahuasca churches today comprised of middle class civil servants who join and actively participate. Many of them are psychotherapists, military personnel, and intellectuals. In these settings, psychotherapeutic and spiritualist approaches are combined with traditional religious doctrines, as these men and women search for spiritual development or self-knowledge. Indeed, on some occasions, drug addicts in search of treatment find their way to ayahuasca rituals.

This trend has taken root in the Peruvian Amazon as well, where a French physician, Jacques Mabit, utilizes the ayahuasca plant in the treatment of drug addicts. We will learn more about this in Chapter 4. Ayahuasca, or hoasca, as it is called in Brazil, is generally used in a religious context. Those who take the tea are effectively using the plant in a controlled environment, making strong statements that nonreligious use is not acceptable.

In Brazil, we see the Roman Catholic Church attempting to maintain hegemony in this very large country. Then, there are the popular religions of African origin, with a number of other positions in between. Brazil has a legacy of racism and slavery of Africans due to the new world slave trade. The Catholicism of the Portuguese colonists in Brazil became a dominant national religion, and powerful landlords helped to maintain it as an official religion. In the eyes of God, everyone, poor and rich, was equal. As time went on, a popular Catholicism emerged, along with Protestant Pentecostal religions. By the 1980s, there was a significant decline in the number of practicing Brazilian Catholics. Scholars writing about Brazilian religions recognize the influence of Kardecism, along with Afro-Brazilian religions such as Candomblé, to be an important ingredient in this religious mix. Where a person resides, and the diverse influences available to him, help Brazilians make their choices of religious affiliation. There is also religious "transit"—with a free acceptance and interchange between different religious systems that both Brazilian and Peruvian citizens are often involved in simultaneously. This can be illustrated by a fieldwork experience that de Rios had in 1967, when she observed an small agricultural village in the north coast of Peru turn out for a parade honoring the Catholic patron saint of the village. Her major informant, a mestizo guide, was driving her to the town of Salas, where a hallucinogenic cactus was to be used that same evening for magical and ritual purposes. In the afternoon the guide, don José, crawled on his knees in humility in the Catholic church to honor the village's patron saint. That same night he also partook of the mescaline cactus brew in a shamanic healing ceremony. Quite a compartmentalization of beliefs!

Those Brazilians who take ayahuasca within a religious context do not disdain the experience or see it simply as "getting high." Rather, for them it is a religious experience encouraged by their designation of ayahuasca as a sacrament. The Portuguese tried to set up a new Portugal in the Brazilian territory that they colonized, and they built a strongly hierarchical society. Over time, general instability developed as more and more people moved away from official Roman Catholic doctrine. In this process, a Dionysian-type religious experience became commonplace, with ecstasy, possession trance, and altered dissociated states becoming valued and sought after within the context of religion. This was done by incorporating music, dance, and movement into rituals, and, in some settings, by taking ayahuasca. Poor people without many resources were still able to negotiate with the spirits and often devoted themselves to becoming followers of a particular spirit entity and propitiating its spiritual forces.

Ayahuasca Use in the Peruvian and Brazilian Amazon

De Rios conducted anthropological fieldwork in the Peruvian Amazon in 1968–1969, 1977, and 1979 on the traditional use of ayahuasca among the urban poor. She traveled through Brazil in 1997 and 1999 to visit UDV temples and work with members of this new religion. In Chapter 5, we will look at the use of ayahuasca within the União do Vegetal Church. Let's turn now to the history of ayahuasca use in the Amazon.

* * *

Ayahuasca is a woody vine comprising species of *Banisteriopsis,* found in the moist tropics of South America. It has been used for its hallucinogenic properties by both native American cultures as well as by mestizos (people of European and native American heritage). Native peoples used ayahuasca for a number of different purposes:[24]

- to obtain divine guidance and to communicate with gods and the spirit world
- to achieve trance states
- to train prospective shamans
- to induce dreams so as to see the future
- for prophecy, as a telepathic agent

- to cure illness through psychic or physical means
- to prevent the malice of others from harming members of the community
- to use visions to prescribe remedies for illness
- to identify an evildoer or agent (witch) responsible for illness

Native peoples believed that spirit forces animate plants and that one can communicate with those forces. They also used the ayahuasca visions to learn when strangers were coming and to know where their enemies were and what plans they had. The plant was used in a ritual manner by shamans. Today, in cities like Iquitos and Pucallpa in Peru, and throughout small villages and towns in Amazonia, there are rural and urban mestizo healers such as the late don Hilde, who use these plants for healing. Let us look at his ayahuasca practice in Pucallpa, Peru and understand his work as a prototypical mestizo healer.

One Mestizo Healer—don Hilde[25]

Traditional healers like don Hilde (who died in 2000) provide as much as 70 percent of the healing available throughout the third world. The use of powerful hallucinogenic plants in such healing endeavors, however, is more limited, although widely found throughout the moist tropics of South America. De Rios visited don Hilde on three occasions in the late 1960s and 1970s. She lived in his clinic and studied his patients, many of whom were given ayahuasca by don Hilde to diagnose and treat witchcraft-derived and physical illness. In her book *Amazon Healer,* de Rios looked at the illnesses treated by the healer as well as at his clients, his plants, and his belief systems.

The most important function of don Hilde's use of ayahuasca was two-fold—in divination, and also retrospectively—to discover the etiology of the illness. Over the centuries, Amazon Indian tribes used these plants for these purposes and to find out the prognosis of illnesses that were believed caused by witchcraft. It was said that witch doctors tried to capture the spirit forces of powerful plants and animals in their environment to mold them to their purposes. With the advent of Christianity and the borrowing of meta-physical beliefs from Europe and the Middle East, a class of individuals called *videntes*[26] (seers) developed on the continent. In Peru, they were called *brujos,* or witches, renowned for their ability to bewitch others by means of their psychic powers. They were said to be able to cause terrible illnesses, misfortunes, and even death to their enemies. The witches prepared hallucinogenic brews made from ayahuasca. They were believed to acquire supernatural power in the form of aid from their animal familiars. The plant tea was used as a diagnostic and revelatory agent. The visions of this LSD-like plant permit the patient to see just what force or individual is believed to be responsible for evildoing. Then, the healer is able to deflect or neutralize the magic that causes the illness and return it to its perpetrator.

Although don Hilde lived in a rapidly changing city with paved roads, automobiles, electricity, telephones, and refrigeration, the vast majority of the urban poor trafficked little (and still do) with these modern conveniences. Their sufferings and lifestyles draw them much closer in experience to the river-edge farmer who ekes out his living in a forest of leeched soils, with droughts and forest burnings all preventing him from realizing more than one or two crop yields per year. The urban dweller's lifestyle at first glance might be indistinguishable from that of the peasant who lives among the numerous riverways outside of Pucallpa, yet both still share deep links with forest aboriginal peoples, especially in their joint concerns about the nature of the moral order—good and evil—and the rampant witchcraft that is believed to infect all areas of social relations.

Traditional Witchcraft Beliefs in the Peruvian Amazon

Peruvian *curanderos* divide illnesses into two groups: those due to natural causes and those due to *daño*, or magical harm or witchcraft. The natural illnesses are caused by the influences of forces of nature and are attributed to distinct elements, in accordance with social and cultural factors. These illnesses lend themselves easily to treatment by Western medicine. Magical illness, however, can only be treated by the curandero, whose mission and mandate is to understand its origin before he can marshal any therapeutic interventions to combat it. For the healer, it does not matter which part of his client's body is afflicted. The illness is believed to derive from interpersonal conflict, and there is no simple set of symptoms to turn to. Urban men and women are consumed by an intense certainty that the envy of their neighbor, relative, or work colleague is responsible for their ailment. Hemorrhages, muscular pain, arthritis, headaches—all can be attributed to envy which inevitably leads to daño. The cause of the illness is more important than the particular way in which the symptoms might appear.

Still another major illness treated by ayahuasca-using mestizo healers is *saladera*.[27] This is a particular cultural disorder which can be understood only in terms of the stresses and strains of culture change, urbanization, and fast-moving modernization facing the Amazonian native. Unlike with other illnesses, which cause physical suffering, patients who came to see mestizo healers like don Hilde about saladera complained only that they had been bewitched and now suffered from misfortune or bad luck. In their words, they were "salted"; everything in life had soured— work, home, a love affair, or relationships with children, spouse, or in-laws. In fact, whatever could possibly go wrong, had gone wrong. The syndrome is an emotional reaction to the breakdown of the family in light of the fast-growing urbanization and its name derives from the Spanish word for salt, *sal.*

Among tropical rain forest farmers who live in cities, the consistent experience of bad luck or generalized misfortune is not perceived as mere chance. On the contrary, people are quick to project their feelings outward toward significant others in their lives, whose malice, envy, or anger they believe is directed against themselves. Malevolent neighbors or work colleagues are identified as the source of, and as being responsible for, this bewitchment. The constant irritation or persistent difficulties encountered in finding a job may not be attributed to a person's own individual inadequacy. Rarely is such failure attributed to abstract economic causes, but rather it is widely attributed to the malice of others. People believe that a number of hexes can cause saladera. For instance, mixing vultures' feces with water and dropping it at someone's doorstep is a sure way to make such misfortunes happen. Salt, when thrown across a neighbor's threshold, or placed on a window sill, is enough provocation for a person to change his residence, since it is believed that catastrophe or death will occur. When salt is placed on living plants, it destroys them. This contrasts with the vital role such a substance has for maintaining health, especially in tropical climates. Thus, salt is both vital and yet feared. It can make life possible, but at the same time it is potentially destructive. Historically salt had an important role in trade, and Campa forest Indians either obtained salt by trade or made long and perilous journeys to the salt mines in the mountains of Chanchamayo, Peru, until they were forcibly stopped from so doing by Peruvian colonists in the nineteenth century. During don Hilde's lifetime, salt taboos were common for individuals who ingested the plant hallucinogen ayahuasca to obtain a vision enabling them to attribute the source of witchcraft to a malevolent individual. The belief is that visionary effects of the drug are enhanced when a person avoids salt.

In areas like Iquitos, salt plays an important role in preservation of meat and fish. Salted foods are an important component of both rural and urban diets, since refrigeration and electricity are costly. Game animals and fish are often retrieved at distances from urban areas and are salted for preservation before being transported to urban centers. When soils yield poorly it is called *salado* ("salted"), indicating the negative role of salt in the agricultural cycle. Linking salt and bad luck can probably be traced to the development of commerce during the colonial period, when the chemical action of salt on containers caused their decay and corroded the metals of transport vessels. From that period onward, salt has found its way into nefarious ingredients making up popular witchcraft hexes which mestizo healers are traditionally called upon to heal. This can include a potion made by women, often prostitutes or women of dubious morality, who collect menstrual blood and other noxious substances that they secretly introduce into a drink. These women delight in breaking up marriages and lure men away from their wives and family. The power attributed to menstrual blood is overwhelming. When de Rios had noisy neighbors in Iquitos in 1968, she was advised to throw coarse salt on their threshold so that they would fear witchcraft hexing and move away!

Mestizo healers spend little time asking about oppressive symptoms. They intuitively know that each human organism will break down in its constituently weak point. They are more concerned to uncover the cause of disharmony in the patient's life before undertaking any real physical therapeutics. Illnesses like daño are believed to be caused by a witch who slips a powerful potion into a drink or throws it across a doorstep late at night. If the witch takes ayahuasca to cause magical harm to his enemy, he uses his psychic powers to bewitch. As with all magical illness that mestizo healers treat, it is imperative that the sick person who suffers from daño should find a healer to neutralize the witch's harm before the illness reaches fatal proportion.

In Peru, we learn that daño's treatment, too, is fundamentally magical. Since it is caused by evil men and women because of envy or other factors, the cure is to liberate the patient from the effects produced by the magic. There are substances that can cause daño when they are imbibed. It can also be introduced by the air or caused by inhalation. Illness can also be caused by elements of nature, such as rivers, mountains and so on. Envy is seen to be omnipresent in social relations, and the malevolence of people can be the enemy. The healer must employ his knowledge to undo his client's damage. The patient is bid to follow his counsel and must alter his relationships with significant others in his environment.

In the tropical rain forest, plants are often believed to possess a mother spirit. By means of *icaros,* or special songs, each curandero has a special set of powers enabling him to heal. Ayahuasca and other hallucinogenic plants have been used to diagnose and achieve revelations. Both the patient and the mestizo healer have these visionary experiences to see the perpetrator of the witchcraft, who appears before them—"seeing is believing." Once the evildoer is identified, the healer's spiritual power is called upon to return the damage to its originator. Only then does the healer seek plant therapeutics to diminish any somatic effects of the illness.

Important to mestizo healing is the fact that the curandero speaks the same language as the patient and is educated in the same society. Healers have tended to be elderly, mature, male, and to appear like parental figures who are kind and generous. They use suggestion, and most of them do short-term crisis intervention. They use behavior modification or adversive conditioning. Certainly there are few psychiatrists or other trained mental health specialists to deal with the onslaught of psychological problems among the urban and rural poor.

The native peoples of the Amazon have a highly developed pharmaco-poeia of medicines and herbs that have been used in healing for many centuries. Mestizo healers have been successful because they treat acute, self-limited disorders, non-life-threatening in nature, and chronic disorders, or somatiza-tions, of minor psychological disorders. Mestizo healers such as don Hilde traditionally render service in a language that the healer and the patient share.

Although there are many materialistic changes in their lives, the belief systems and concerns about the moral order, the nature of good and evil, and witchcraft beliefs are very much alive. De Rios in 2007 was able to briefly interview one mestizo healer who had worked with don Hilde before his death, who was very angry at the changes he saw all around him. Healing was no longer linked to a philosophy of good and evil, witchcraft and healing. Neo-shamans were taking over and destroying the traditional field of mestizo healing.

Such urban mestizo healers today have lost the respect of their own com-munity. Those like don Hilde exercise little formal power in terms of social control of the community. Don Hilde functioned to protect his client in a personal way. In the past, witchcraft accusations may have been rampant, and witches were hunted down and destroyed, even in Pucallpa. Few people today openly confront their enemies or make accusation against them. In the past, only shamans who possessed special powers were able to see spirits in their human forms. Animal familiars of the shaman were good spirits who assumed the guise of certain species of birds and animals. The shaman was able to call upon the spirits of plants such as ayahuasca and tobacco when they were needed. In the past, the mestizo shaman would access mind-altering LSD-like plants such as ayahuasca and *toé*, which he would brew for several hours. These vision-inducing plants would be given to the sick person and that person would try to see the individual responsible for the troubling illness or misfortune. The term "retrocognition" is useful here, as the ayahuasca visions would enable the healer to see back in time to the moment of his client's bewitchment and identify the guilty party. Then his job was to turn the evil back to its perpetrator.

It is true that urban healers have lost many of the shamanic elements of their Amazonian forebears. Few women practice the healing arts. Those who do, until recent years, were more likely to prepare abortion-inducing drugs, or *pusangas*—love potions—to enable their clients to bewitch a paramour or ex-suitor. The general belief was that when women were still menstruating, they would be considered to be polluters and not have access to healing spirits until they reached menopause. In Amazonia, this theme is consistent with the taboos which limit the activities of menstruating women, derived from prehistoric tribal times. The power attributed to menstrual blood is interesting and taboos exist which restrict women from entering the forest to gather plants during this time of the month. Neither can they weed gardens or travel on the rivers. In 1968, de Rios and a student assistant were both in a canoe that almost capsized as they went to visit a family in an outlying island near Iquitos. The near-capsizing of the boat was attributed by the family they visited to the fact that the student assistant was menstruating and offending the spirits of the river!

There is a rich belief system among peasants in cities like Iquitos and Pucallpa concerning love in general, and its persistence. Amazonian men have historically had the reputation of a philandering lifestyle, establishing families in different cities as they traveled for trade and commerce. In fact, regarding the type of love and affection that is natural and spontaneous—this type of love is believed not to endure. It is only *amor cochinado* ("piggy" love) due to the action of a charm or witchcraft pusanga (potion) that is thought to be the most durable. Often women who suffer from saladera have been abandoned by their husbands or common-law companions. They seek help from mestizo healers who, they believe, while under the influence of ayahuasca will be able to draw their husbands back to their sides. When de Rios studied don Hilde's activities in 1977, as many as one in four adult patients in his clinic sought help for this problem. Unlike daño, where a third party, a witch, is brought into the picture, saladera is a direct witchcraft activity practiced by one's enemy, who may personally prepare a hex pusanga. Occasionally, new clients of don Hilde asked him to perform witchcraft upon a recalcitrant spouse or boyfriend, which he generally refused to do.

In his urban practice don Hilde reflected only minimally the heritage of the tribal shaman. He was Christian, although he was not a practicing Catholic or Protestant. He was a member of one of the spiritualist mystical-philosophical groups in the region. He lived in a community where much of Indian lore has been forgotten, but a fierce belief in spirit forces still pervades the urban community. Don Hilde's beliefs in spiritualism interfaced neatly with aboriginal ones. The common knowledge of the effects of healing plants are less and less generally known in cities like Pucallpa. Many mestizo ayahuasca healers, however, continue to believe that they control the spirit of the plants they use, and that they will transform into noble beasts of the forests, like jaguars or eagles. Both healer and client share perceptions of a world of spiritual animation concordant with the region's historical pattern, despite massive culture changes—the belief that the misfortunes over which poor people lack control can be righted by spiritual intervention. The moral order has meaning. Today, urban mestizo healers like don Hilde respond to the amoralism of the city, focusing on problems of drug abuse, prostitution, family breakdown and child or wife abuse. When the healer has rectitude, he is protected by spirits and is able to transform the spirit world to serve his clients. This is congruent with ancient Amazonian patterns. The healing of don Hilde certainly differed in kind and substance both from orthodox medical techniques available in the city and from the neo-shamans we will visit in this book.

More on don Hilde's Techniques

Don Hilde was a specialist in the use of ayahuasca. He would take the plant himself and only gave it to patients whose illnesses had not advanced sufficiently to cause them discomfort. This was due to its strong purgative effect. During the time that don Hilde was under the influence of ayahuasca, he would see the individual responsible for bewitching his client appearing before him in a vision. Drawing on his own personal power (and shamanism is all about personal power), he would be able to nullify the witch's nefarious activities and return his patient to good health. He would also have visions about which herbal preparations he would need to give his patient to treat the presenting illness. This traditional urban mestizo use of ayahuasca is quite different from the way in which the UDV, for example, incorporates the tea into its Christian and African-derived belief systems.

Don Hilde personified the typical ayahuasca healer of the 1960s and 1970s. From early morning to late at night, living in a large, eight-room wooden shack with no running water or electricity, don Hilde would see men, women, and children who sought his help—people from all over the city, as well as from distant hamlets a few hours away by bus or boat. They waited patiently in the *sala,* a large, bare room with benches set against the walls. The first patients came at daybreak, almost always women with their sick children. Upon rising, don Hilde checked out the supply of plant medicines he had on hand in his consulting room, a tiny curtained place where he met his patients, which was equipped with two chairs and a table that was cluttered with bottles and herbs. He was a master herbalist. He read fortune-telling cards called *naipes,* when asked to, and the fortune-telling cards enabled him to isolate stressors in the client's milieu.

In the course of an average day, don Hilde saw as many as 25 patients, many with their young babies or small children. He was clearly a local practitioner, appreciated by the community for his abilities and skills in counseling, for his knowledge of plant medicines, and for his access to spiritual realms. His fees took the form of donations, and were not according to any payment schedule. Seventy percent of his patients had also visited medical doctors during the previous year.

Many more women than men consulted the healer. Over half of his clients were young children suffering from the ravages of malnutrition and the host of diseases associated with third world poverty. Adults came with tales of misfortune and bad luck—the saladera complex of the region discussed earlier, which don Hilde treated with spiritual solace, herbal teas, midnight baths, and his own source of energy. Others suffered from bodily ailments exacerbated by the stress of poverty, unemployment, malnutrition, and overcrowding. Some suffered from the results of moral anguish, being fearful of bewitchment caused by those in the community who disliked them, who despised them, or who wished to humble them. Don Hilde accepted all who came to his door. Each patient averaged two or three visits. Many of don Hilde's patients had access to cosmopolitan medicine in the two major regional hospitals or in smaller medical clinics or offices of private practitioners.

Don Hilde was slender and of average height. Born in 1917 in a small hamlet near Pucallpa, he was a mestizo, heir to Spanish and Indian racial mixture in South America over the last 400 years. His parents were poor farmers. He attended public school for only three years and worked at odd jobs to earn money. He married and settled in the central Amazon city of Pucallpa, where he worked as a carpenter. While still an adolescent, he had visions of Christian saints, but he did not recognize his ability to heal people until he was well established in his carpentry trade and had become a family man with three children. From time to time, he treated a few patients in his home while continuing his commercial activities. With the spread of his reputation for successful healing over the years, he devoted more and more time to curing. He began to use the plant hallucinogen ayahuasca and read books on hypnosis. He tried to induce trance-like states in himself.

Healers like don Hilde have complex philosophical or mystical systems that they study and follow, but such doctrines are not widely held among their clients. The healer and his clients just do not share the healer's esoteric knowledge. Community harmony and cohesion are nonexistent in the city, where social change has proceeded for almost 400 years. The native Amazonian resident has been wrenched out of his tribal lifestyle. The materialistic focus of modern medicine, with its belief in the body as a machine, something which breaks down and must be repaired, is not harmonic with the beliefs of urban peasants, whose world of spirits endures despite all the changes that have occurred in their lives.

Herbal lore of plant medicines has become less and less generally known in cities like Pucallpa and Iquitos. Only a few who take the trouble to learn, like don Hilde, now know what was common knowledge in past times. The aspect of the animal familiar has lost some of its historic traditions in urban healing with the influence of Christianity, and concepts borrowed from scientific vocabularies in the mass media replace in some people the ancient belief systems.

The old-time shamanic role has been stripped of its social control mechanism. No longer do adult men and women function to protect the community from its enemies. The state has to be dealt with—the natural government, including police, bureaucracy, social services, the Western medical establishment, and so on. All the mestizo shaman qua urban healer can now offer his client is to protect him or her—protect from the evil that everyone knows is omnipresent and which threatens everyone's well-being. Don Hilde's beliefs in spiritualism interfaced nicely with aboriginal ones. His clients may not have comprehended very well the subtle and complex philosophical system that he would articulate when asked. But both he and his client shared perceptions of a world of spiritual animation concordant with the region's historical pattern, despite the massive culture changes. Even though many of don Hilde's patients had a primary school education, they suffered from the despair of the urban poor everywhere. They found reaffirmation in the healer's ability to redress the evil they saw all around them. Don Hilde and others like him were able to arbitrate the upheavals in their clients' social relations. The misfortunes over which poor people lack control can be righted by spiritual intervention. Alienation can be distanced, and the moral order has meaning. Today, healers like don Hilde respond to moral breakdown in the city, to problems of drug abuse, prostitution, family disintegration, and child and wife abuse. The healer's rectitude, his protection by the spirits, and his ability to transform the spirit world to serve his clients are all congruent with ancient Amazonian patterns. When asked, don Hilde cited his success as due to his involvement with a mystical-philosophical group called *Septrionism de la Amazonia,* which he joined in 1974 as it organized in Pucallpa. In the group's name he established a large center for healing in the outskirts of the city.

Septrionism of the Amazon

Septrionism is both a mystical and a philosophical doctrine, established in 1968 by Claudio Cedeño and his wife, Placy Gonzales. It was originally known as Amazonian Brahmanism-Lamaism. The source of knowledge that gave rise to Septrionism and its doctrines was communicated to Brother Claudio in revelations—in the form of ideas, norms, plans, and fundamentals—with the purpose of achieving coherence and unity between religious and moral values, as well as with science. There are laws of causality and reality that face human beings; such laws deal with people's missions in society and the harmony between science and religion. Human tribulation—suffering and affliction—has sociopolitical causes that human beings can overcome to achieve spiritual peace.

Deity is conceptualized as the Eon of Eternal Intelligence, with God represented not as a being, but as a conjunct of energies. The Eon of Eternal Intelligence functionally is the Creator and is constituted as Energy. Man is a dual being with an astral-atomic spirit and body. The goal of the organization is to dignify human beings, to make them understand their reality. It tries to harmonize human interests, in the hope that man can live in peace and in accord with society. The group reconciles mysticism with the scientific aspect of human culture. Humans are made to comprehend that their instinctive nature is the cause of their passions and their tribulations, and that until a person rationally uses his intelligence, he or she will experience conflicts and suffering. Eclectic in nature, its beliefs are that whatever religion or creed a person professes, as long as it reveres the father and his creation, that person is on the correct path. Religion to the Septrionics is not a divine mandate but a human spiritual need, providing a way for mankind to identify himself with the Creator. Septrionics worship not messengers sent by the Creator but the Creator exclusively. They do glorify all the messengers or prophets who have given rise to the different religions of the world.

Don Hilde drew upon the constant and continuing help of a spirit guide, under whose protection he was placed when he joined the group. The beliefs of Septrionism are complex and merit their own book to present the beliefs and rituals. Such a focus on esoterism and mysticism is not at all uncommon among traditional mestizo healers. Don Hilde eventually began to use ayahuasca less and less, depending more upon his innate visionary abilities to diagnose and heal the illnesses that his patients suffered.

Like many ayahuasca healers, when don Hilde first interviewed a patient in the small and cramped cubbyhole adjoining his waiting room, he took his or her pulse. Like his shamanic forebears, don Hilde did not question a patient about symptoms, but rather he concentrated intensely as his hand passes over the patient's head, to read what he termed the "electromagnetic energies" of the client. This enabled don Hilde to understand if the illness was a natural one or was related to witchcraft. Spontaneously he entered into an altered state of consciousness to receive visionary input. Further diagnostic insights came to him during ayahuasca sessions, which he conducted three or four times a week, generally on Tuesdays, Fridays, or Saturdays. Every few weeks or so, don Hilde disappeared for the day with his machete and a large jute sack. He put on his sturdy walking boots and went to the forest outskirts of Pucallpa, near a large lagoon, to gather medicinal plants. He brought the herbs home and prepared his medicines, until the supply dwindled and he had to repeat the process. He had great rapport with his patients and commanded their trust and respect. Over the years, he accumulated many successes in treating a variety of illness. This is an area of the world where widespread beliefs in witchcraft still abound, which causes people to be fearful, angry, enraged, and to feel helpless. Their faith in the power of healers like don Hilde permits their fears to fade away, so that they can maintain some kind of emotional equilibrium. At don Hilde's death, two buses full of his former patients and friends went to the cemetery to honor him at his burial!

Manuel Cordova-Rios—A Famous Ayahuasquero in Iquitos, Peru[28]

This well-known ayahuasca healer lived from 1887–1978 and is perhaps the most famous mestizo shaman who has lived in the Amazon. He was born in Iquitos, and as a child, he helped his parents in the extraction of rubber from trees in the forest. He was captured by the Amahuaca Indians, and their leader, Chumo, tried to make him into a powerful shaman and tribal headman, since as a mestizo he had access to knowledge and secrets of the firearms that mestizos and whites used to control and dominate the Indians.

Chumo and other Amahuaca shamans transmitted to Cordova-Rios knowledge of the black panther, which they called *Ino Moxo,* and they renamed Manuel for this powerful animal. They taught him all the secrets of ayahuasca use. He became a powerful shaman who took ayahuasca supposedly more than 500 times. In the height of his power, Cordova-Rios decided to return to the urban mestizo world that he remembered from his childhood. He fled and arrived in Iquitos and experienced a large number of changes in his life. Thanks to his extraordinary knowledge about the forest, medicinal plants, and in particular, ayahuasca, Cordova-Rios was contracted to be a forest guide of an American firm, Astoria Manufacturing Company, located in Iquitos since 1918. Astoria was dedicated to exporting forest animal species and fine woods to the United States, in particular, mahogany and cedar. He gained fame as one of the most accomplished shamans in Iquitos in the 1960s up to the 1970s. In this time, Cordova-Rios was one of the few mestizo shamans in the city. At the beginning of the twentieth century, shamanism and folk healing were practiced by indigenous peoples—almost clandestinely, in the rural zones among small river-edge towns. If an indigenous person practiced shamanism in the city, it was done in the periphery, in marginal zones where the poor habitually lived. Indigenous people were and continue to be the poorest among the poor.

After the mid-century, and into the 1960s, there was a process of rural migration to the cities of Iquitos, Pucallpa, Requena, Yurimaguas, and others, and the first mestizo shamans appeared, in competition with their few indigenous colleagues. Cordova-Rios lived long years in a street called Huallaga in Iquitos. Rumrrill visited with him several times. His life was made famous due to the biographies written about him by the American F. Bruce Lamb, particularly his book *Wizard of the Upper Amazon.* Cordova-Rios had prestige among medical and scientific specialists in Iquitos as well. In one interview with the world-famous Peruvian psychiatrist Carlos Alberto Seguin, Cordova-Rios described his healing techniques and medicines. Then, as he got up abruptly to leave, he said to Rumrrill and Seguin, "No me crees: es pura mentira"—Don't believe me, it's all a lie!

In another interview with Rumrrill, they sat in Cordova-Rios' front room to talk about the patients who sought out don Manuel incessantly from the morning to the evening. While there, Rumrrill heard someone knock loudly at the door. Don Manuel was smoking his shaman's pipe and only reluctantly went to open the door. He asked the visitor, Ruben: "What do you want?" Ruben told him that he desperately needed Manuel to cure him, that he was very sick. In Rumrrill's eye, the patient seemed ill, pale, and weak. Cordova-Rios looked Ruben over and told him to return in 15 days, effectively kicking the man out of his house. Rumrrill asked Cordova-Rios why he treated the sick man so badly. Cordova-Rios looked at Rumrrill fixedly and said: "I have just looked at his interior and I have seen that he is going to die in 15 days. It is too late for me to do anything for him."

Patients came from all over, even overseas, to be treated by don Manuel. On another occasion, when Rumrrill accompanied an acquaintance to visit Cordova-Rios, the man recited a liturgy of bodily aches, pains, and diseases he suffered. Time after time, the curandero went to a room in his house full of small bottles—different colored roots and fruits hanging in bottles on the wall—all medicinal produce of Amazon flora and fauna. The patient took each remedy—one for ulcers, one for each illness discussed, some quite rare. Finally he had in his hands more than a dozen bottles to cure him, even one for saladera. Rumrrill's friend left the house happy and content that all his earthly illnesses and bad luck were things of the past. Unlike other mestizo healers, including don Hilde, Manuel Cordova-Rios did not look into the patient's future by means of fortune-telling cards.

Fortune-Telling Cards as a Diagnostic Technique[29]

During her fieldwork in Iquitos, de Rios came across the *naipes*— fortune-telling cards used as a technique to obtain data among urban peasants living in the squatter settlement of Belen in Iquitos. Eventually she became a *curiosa,* a person who used these cards for men and women in the community, who would pay her a small fee for the service (the money thus obtained was spent on medicines given back to sick people in the community).

The naipes accompany ayahuasca as one more technique used among the urban poor to divine the future. Early ethnographic reports show Amazon peasants using these cards to foretell the future and to find out the prognosis of illnesses believed due to witchcraft. The individual vidente, or seer, developed everywhere on the South American continent.

The naipes were used by don Hilde when requested by his clients. De Rios inadvertently fell into the role of fortune-teller when she lived in Iquitos from 1968–1969. One can see how the suggestibility properties of the cards enhanced the power of a shaman healer like don Hilde. De Rios learned to use the naipes deck in 1967 on her first trip to Peru and observed coastal healers using this technique in preparation for a San Pedro mescaline cactus drink in a healing setting. When she spent a year in the rain forest and became a curiosa (someone who knows things), she kept careful notes of her readings. When she analyzed the naipes' structure at a later point, it was clear that there was a type of grammar or symbology connected to these ancient cards, which were brought to Latin America by priests in the sixteenth century for purposes of gaming. They became incorporated into healing techniques over the centuries. When de Rios began to accept small amounts of money for the service, her practice expanded dramatically, as only an intern tells fortunes for free.

A certain amount of skill is required to take discrete items associated with each card and turn them into a story, so that three or four cards read together present a short narrative. A book by Madame LeNormand, reputed to be Napoleon's adviser, helps the novice to learn how to read the cards. After the reading, clients can ask three questions of the cards, about anything they wish, with a "yes" or "no" answer possible if a good luck card turned up, for example, one up, one down. These cards can be traced to tenth century

China and appear in the fourteenth century in several European countries, including Italy, Germany, and Spain. Originally tarot cards were linked to the esoteric Jewish Kabbalah tradition, which had 22 tarot cards relating to the letters of the Hebrew alphabet. The cards used by the French for divination were derived from tarot cards and were called Naibi. The term comes from the Arab *naib,* "he who represents," or "he who plays." The deck consists of 48 cards, with nine number cards and three figure cards in four different suits. De Rios was able to see how six cards were classified as signifying outright misfortune such as business loss, false pregnancy, etc. Another 11 cards also signify misfortune. Throughout the reading, the fortune-teller strives to connect the client's interests to the cards' significance. The patient is encouraged to talk during the card reading, and this helps the healer identify interpersonal tensions, anxieties, and conflicts that can contribute to illness. Misfortune cards occur in very high frequency in a given reading, enabling the healer to probe and gain insight into the client's problems. These cards are a stimulus to help both the healer and the client understand the messages in the card reading. The individual responds to suggested communications without a critical examination of his or her judgments, opinions, attitudes, or patterns of behavior. The cards certainly helped don Hilde to provide his client with a sense of his own omnipotence—which would be marshaled to help the client recover from illness, as he or she gained faith in the healer's abilities.

Don Hilde's Patients—A Cross-Section

When we turn to discussing the drug tourists in Chapter 4, it will seem like we are on a different planet, with regard to the change in venue of the mostly mestizo healers who have become neo-shamans for the cash cow of visitors they anticipate and seek. It is helpful to see what the clients of traditional mestizo healers like don Hilde look like, in order to understand how totally unprepared this mestizo population is to heal the New Age tourists who come looking for spiritual help and redemption.

In 1977, de Rios moved into don Hilde's clinic for the month of February and interviewed the entire patient population that came for diagnosis and treatment during that period of time. Given the sort of primary health care available in underdeveloped countries like Peru, the folk healer such as don Hilde is a jack-of-all-trades, a prototypical generalist practitioner. Don Hilde saw all kinds of patients—from the very young to those destined in Western society for the psychologist, the orthopedic surgeon, or the psychiatrist. He was, in fact, the epitome of a primary care physician. In a single day he could give seven enemas to young children, advise mothers on their children's remedies, brew herbal teas for some, prepare herbal medicines for others, read the naipes, counsel a businessman about a decision to make, and so on. The healer has links to spiritual realms that prepare him for a diverse number of tasks. We wonder how someone like don Hilde managed not to suffer burn-out nor have his energies drained by the onslaught of patients who visited him on a daily basis. He claimed that he drew energy from a source greater than himself, energy that was channeled through him.

Some clients were so ill that they could not come to his clinic themselves. They might send a grandchild or son in their place. A large percentage of the clients had consulted medical doctors in Pucallpa over the previous six months before seeing don Hilde. De Rios interviewed 96 patients of his during February 1977. Seventy presented with a physical ailment that they could describe, if questioned. Another 26 came without any physical symptoms but secure in their knowledge that they needed help for bewitchment, or that they suffered from bad fortune, or they sometimes wanted advice about the future. Don Hilde reported that 62 percent of his clients had natural illnesses, while the remainder suffered from nonnatural disorders directly related to the evil malice of others. Illnesses directly related to witchcraft were found among another 25 patients. Still another 11 clients had disorders considered to be psychological in nature. Most of the clients had attended high school, though 11 of the 96 adults only attended elementary school. A few had some additional technical education. In the course of a month, don Hilde saw 38 new patients, and each client averaged three visits. Almost one third of his clients had a personal experience with ayahuasca. Certainly most of them had a relative or friend who took the purge to diagnose witchcraft-related illness. Those under 30 years of age had less knowledge of the drug, and in 1992, it appeared that ayahuasca use was diminishing. More men than women used ayahuasca. Two young men habitually smoked cocaine paste and were brought to don Hilde by their parents, in the hopes that they would be able to stop their constant stealing to support the drug habit. Two women wanted don Hilde to bewitch their lovers so they would marry them.

Fifty-one of the clients were young children, four of whom suffered from witchcraft disease believed caused by their parents' enemies. Don Hilde saw many of these illnesses as recent onset, while others were more chronic in nature. Clients' marriages were quite stable, and most of don Hilde's patients lived with their spouses. Women had some work out of the house on farms, or in markets, selling or peddling goods; or working as cooks, laundresses, or seamstresses. Men worked in laboring jobs on a day-to-day basis with little economic stability.

Unlike the neo-shamans we will see in Chapter 4, don Hilde did not advertise his services, and his clients learned about his clinic from recommendations of former patients, or relatives, friends, or neighbors. Most of the men did not see physicians before coming to see don Hilde, while women usually did have that experience. Many more women than men believed in witchcraft in their own lives or that of relatives. Older women reported that they had personally experienced witchcraft in their lifetimes, causing them misery and causing their children or loved ones to die, which made their marriages split apart. Those believing they were bewitched kept secret about their seeking help. Don Hilde's fees were quite reasonable, and he accepted donations far below that charged by a medical doctor in the city. Moreover, his fee also included medicines, quite distinct from the medical establishment.

Most of the adults that visited don Hilde had some education and the vast majority finished 6 years of elementary school. Married adults comprised a stable group who lived with their spouses. Most clients fit into a middle range of occupations and income levels in Pucallpa, with laborers, peddlers, domestics, small-scale wholesalers, independent workers, and urban artisans most representative. Traditional healers like don Hilde generally would obtain their patients from personal referrals, and almost all 96 clients interviewed by de Rios were at his clinic on the personal recommendation of a friend or relative who said they had been cured themselves, and who accompanied the patient the first time. A considerable part of don Hilde's practice was comprised of patients who suffered from witchcraft diseases. Case after case recounted the envy, greed, anger, or vengeance that motivated people to personally prepare evil potions to cause harm to the patients. Witchcraft beliefs, interestingly enough, have not given way in the face of rapid culture change. Witchcraft fears and secretiveness were present, creating still another climate of anxiety in addition to the day-to-day problems of people who suffered somatic discomforts. This anxiety only intensified the illnesses, provoking insomnia, further depressing low energy levels, and presenting problems in coping. Don Hilde's calming teas, his sanctity and simplicity, his meditation ceremonies once a week, and his antianxiety purges like ayahuasca, his low fees, and his obvious concern give rise for a successful therapeutic milieu.

Don Hilde clearly practiced a short-term, crisis-oriented form of healing. Both don Hilde and his clients accepted the existence and effectiveness of witches; they each believed that evil is rampant on earth, and they agreed that there is a need to neutralize, annul, and mitigate its power and effect.

Don Hilde and the Paranormal

In urban and rural areas of the Amazon, most people are convinced that individual psychic powers are present everywhere, and that they can be manipulated by people—either to harm one's enemy, or to heal an illness. The world of illness divides into two types: natural and supernatural. The role of a traditional folk healer like don Hilde is to determine if an illness is caused by the psychic powers or sorcery of another person. Witches are known as evil men and women who, for a fee paid in advance, will wreak vengeance on someone's enemies. Ayahuasca healers poise themselves to find out what the problem is, where the envy emanated, who wants vengeance, or who holds rancor or other strong negative emotions toward the client. Witches are believed to cause misfortune by means of their psychic power, and healers can counter this by use of their own considerable forces to neutralize the evil and rectify the client's problems. Scientists deny the validity of such beliefs, and sociologically-oriented investigators try to tie these beliefs in with politics or other psychological explanations.

Don Hilde had a strong reputation as a seer. He was not a trickster, and he had no agents in the community listening to the tales of woe and reporting back to him, to startle his client with unusual feats of mentalism like a nightclub performer. Pucallpa was and is just too geographically spread out and populous for that kind of trickery to work—it is a fast-changing urban environment where neighborhoods are constantly being reconstituted as people come and go. Plant drugs like ayahuasca are important whenever social stresses exist, because culturally they have been used for their visionary properties to provide retrocognitive and purportedly accurate information directly from the client's past. This permits the patient, the healer, or both to ascertain in their own minds who is the evildoer responsible for bewitching the patient. As don Hilde described the reading he obtained from a client, he would put his finger on a particular stressful situation contributing to the person's illness. His reputation would be clearly enhanced in the process. This strong emotional impact, plus the purgative, antianxiety effects of the ayahuasca, put to shame any Western doctor's technique. Mestizo healers like don Hilde maintain absolute anonymity within their clinics. There are no records, no names asked, no medical history taken. The force of the seer's ability to tell the patient what is troubling him, in reasonably explicit terms, must create a sense of intimacy and what psychoanalysts call a strong transference effect. On subsequent visits, patients have brought along friends and relatives to be helped, much as they themselves were.

This ability to divine the future impresses upon the patient that the healer can control natural and supernatural forces. When a patient transgresses the community's moral system, he may assume that the healer is also powerful enough to grant him absolution before the spirit world, given the healer's prior knowledge of drug or alcohol abuse or other immoral behavior. His own guilt is easier to handle. There is a high degree of suggestibility that arises from the perceived omnipotence of the healer as he deals with the spirit world. In this sense, it is very common in Peru where a client and therapist share the same basic assumptions when it comes to dealing with the world of spirit. Don Hilde's esoteric knowledge was in demand. The healer is supposed to impart knowledge to his patient. Only an intern-novice, not a fully competent healer, would ask questions. Don Hilde's intake procedure was one of telling, not of asking. What really matters here is not the veracity of the paranormal communications between healers like don Hilde and their clients. The healers in mestizo life are sought out by patients because of their reputed vidente qualities and abilities. These are then reaffirmed in the lives of the patients through the healer's performance. In this shared assumptive world of healer and client, there will be a feedback into biochemical and hormonal processes. Instead of asking the questions "does telepathy work? And if so, how?" rather we should focus on whether these beliefs exist. Is a symbolic environment created, one where the healer's communication with his patient can transfer the healing to the patient's "doctor within" and marshal those tools that enhance natural healing?

Conversations with don Hilde

In 1977, de Rios interviewed don Hilde about his beliefs regarding the ayahuasca work he did. He said that when his clients' illnesses were natural, he felt different from when they were caused by a witchcraft hex. He felt the illness as an exaggerated force of energy like shock waves and the body vibrates. He said that when drugs like ayahuasca are used carelessly, the colors and visionary forms prevent a person from seeing, and the drug actually gets in the way of the visionary effect. He avoided spiritism, which in his opinion was access to lower spirit forms. He believed firmly that one must be spiritually dominant and have access only to higher spiritual forces. Don Hilde talked about *aliados,* spirit allies that animate the healing plants. He said that good men and women try only to heal. Thus the ally is an entity that a person has to dominate. Without a teacher one cannot learn how to do this, and those who depend entirely on the ayahuasca plant do not learn anything else. Special preparatory diets are falling out of interest, and there are few people around who go off to the virgin forest and live on handfuls of food. Few take different plants to learn their effects while fastidiously controlling their diets. Each plant has its limited power.

Don Hilde stated that no woman can become a healer while young, because of the power of her menstrual blood, which negates any spiritual force of power; also, the force of that blood can only destroy, not heal. Apprentices have to stay away from the power of menstruating women during their training. Once a woman reaches menopause, she can become an ayahuasca healer but has to go alone to the forest to control her food intake and learn from the plants. Many women become witches, according to don Hilde, to gain money by doing bad things. They prepare *cochinados*— "piggish" hexes—for a price, to cause harm to others.

During ayahuasca ceremonies, don Hilde would concentrate intently on each person. He saw each body as if under X-ray scrutiny, commenting out loud on what each one suffered. He would see a thorn that was introduced into the body by a witch. The patient would experience the thorn like a real thing causing pain, even though don Hilde said it was symbolic. Evil witches can cause illness in as little as 24 hours. Some cause death and bewitch for the sheer pleasure of exercising their power. During an ayahuasca session, forces of evil are present in the room, and the healer feels the desperation of patients everywhere. A wise healer has to have his own defenses—good forces that hover around him. The session is like a battlefield, and one can easily become sick. Before medicines can be used, the healer has to eliminate the hex. Don Hilde said he did not talk about fees to his patients. After they received their medicine they generally asked about fees. He answered that he wanted to see them well. He did not think in terms of money, nor did he aspire to great ambitions. Since he did not charge for his service but accepted donations, he had little problems with authorities.

Don Hilde did not limit himself to only one kind of problem but focused on the spiritual aspects of the patient's life. He did not ask patients questions about their symptoms. He would look and think. He would connect spiritually with the patient's body to see where the pain was that was bothering each. He would take his or her illness into his body through his empathy, and then he was able to diagnose. He then found a medicine that corresponded to that illness.

He also acknowledged that there were few good apprentices willing to work hard and to learn. Some would only learn through talking. Some would provoke the maestro, and fighting began. Some were interested only in money, to gain the favors of women, and to learn to be ayahuasqueros to attract women to their beds. He complained about apprentices who, after a couple of weeks, thought they knew everything.

Don Hilde depended more on energies than icaros. He said that each plant has its own icaro, to put the person in touch with the healing spirits of that plant. When one takes ayahuasca or other plants, one learns the songs spontaneously. Don Hilde used the ayahuasca only once a week. His work was observation, compared with healers who use ayahuasca depending on the revelations. Many of them are involved with reprisal to harm their clients' enemies. Don Hilde was also a firm believer in remembering dreams as part of self-development, to help with mental development—one can receive instruction through dreams. His visions helped him know which pharmaceutical medicines to use.

Urban Indigenous Healers: The Shipibo: don Guillermo Arrévalo and His Center, "Espíritu de Anaconda"[30]

One contemporary Shipibo healer, don Guillermo Arrévalo, is in practice in Iquitos today. Arrévalo's career is hardly the usual indigenous or mestizo biography. Arrévalo started his work as a curandero after completing a university degree in pharmacy at the age of 24. He has about 35 years of work already under his belt. His healing center is located along the highway from Iquitos, Peru to Nauta and was named after a small stream; it bears the name "anaconda," which is the largest snake in the world. In the view of the indigenous Indians of the Amazon, this snake is a powerful protective totem. It is found in the serpentine rivers of the area. The Pano Indians of this region believed the anaconda to be a totem that helps fishermen to find schools of fish.

In Arrévalo's center, the communal indigenous houses, called *malocas,* have thatched roofs and wooden construction. All the habitations of the center are constructed in a very unusual forest—a forest of slim rods. The species of trees in this forest are quite narrow in comparison with other tropical forests that exist elsewhere. These slim forest species are only found in sandy dirt of ancient marine origin, such as occurs among certain Amazon soils. These trees cannot hide or sustain birds, large monkeys, or other species of wild animals that live in forests of large trees with abundant food resources.

The first impression that a visitor has, arriving at the Espíritu de Anaconda Center, is that he is entering a park. As the visitor begins his walk around the malocas, accompanied by don Guillermo or his wife, Sonia, the charm of the site takes over. The healer is a small man, around 60 years old. He speaks with a soft and deep voice. His knowledge of Amazonian nature, and the properties and curative principles of the plants, are overwhelming. He claims to know the properties of more than 2,000 plants. For him the forest is an open book that is a privilege to read—a privilege only for those who are capable of dialoguing with sacred plants, with the mother of the plants, ayahuasca.

Whoever arrives to submerge himself in the secrets of the Amazonian world, and in the profundities of his own self, by ingesting the purge ayahuasca finds that the Anaconda Center offers him the ideal atmosphere and setting to do so. The birds sing, the wind whips through the forest, time appears to stand still, and the branches of the delicate trees make a whistling sound. The meals are vegetarian, and everything is to build up to the event of taking the ayahuasca. Don Guillermo's knowledge and wisdom derives from centuries and many generations of curanderos who constructed the shamanic system that he uses. When night falls, with the ayahuasca drink in hand that was carefully prepared all day long, and keeping to a diet that restricts salt, chiles, and lard, those persons who are going to follow the diet are sent to a nearby maloca in the midst of the night. One hears only breathing and the sound of hearts beating and the song of the owl in the darkness of the night. Once the voyage begins, all those present are seated in a circle. Don Guillermo begins to sing his icaros in a deep voice, persuasive and mysterious. There are songs that break up out of the depths of his soul and the mystery of the jungle. He offers the drink to the participants, as he smokes tobacco from his shamanic pipe and blows the smoke over the cup being offered to his patient. This evokes the spirit force that he controls to help in his healing activities. A few minutes later, which appears to be an eternity for some of the patients, visions emerge from an inaccessible depth, from an unfathomable abyss. Each one travels to the end of himself in a voyage that is marvellous and revealing, leading inevitably and inexorably to his own destiny.

On average, Arrévalo usually sees 10–12 visitors at a time who come to him for a treatment of three weeks' duration. He does not accept tourists who come only for the recreational aspect of the ceremony. About half of the visitors suffer from depression, bulimia, or some other psychiatric disorder. The rest are there to learn. Some even choose a full-scale apprenticeship, pledging to stay at least two years and undergo various dietary and lifestyle restrictions. Overall, Arrévalo's patients come with very few complaints of physical ailments.

In a recent visit, those working with Arrévalo were all foreigners, which is generally the case in this center. Without doubt, the cost is too high for Peruvians, ranging from $40–50 a day for foreigners, and only a little less for the locals. This came home to de Rios in 1972, when a friend in Peru tried to visit a famous shaman in the coastal area of Trujillo, whose charges to treat a culture-specific illness called *susto* (fright) was more costly than a consultation with a neurosurgeon in Lima!

Arrévalo holds a ceremony every night but invites visitors every other night. He discusses the changes in each person's health profile individually and in groups. Both the individual and group discussions are very similar to the "traditional" American psychotherapy interaction. During the discussions,

Arrévalo emphasizes the need of the patient to be actively engaged in the healing process; forgiveness, compassion, and self-esteem were also themes that he focused upon.

The healer modifies the ayahuasca dose in accordance with the condition of the patient and any previous reactions to the brew he or she might have had. If the reaction has been exceptionally strong, Arrévalo prescribes a spoonful every day for about a week prior to the ceremony. He also practices different diets. In the afternoon before one ceremony, a patient has to take a vomitive. If a patient has a "genetic problem," then Arrévalo immediately refuses to work with the patient and sends him or her to a local hospital.

All patients who were there for treatment claimed that their condition significantly improved as early as halfway through the treatment. They all mentioned the compassion, love, and guidance of the healer, their improved self-esteem, and various kinds of spiritual discoveries they associated with accepting their own strengths and weaknesses.

During the discussions with patients, Guillermo does not share details of curing, or the structure of the spirit world. Clients are simply not given detailed information. However, this is exactly what he discusses at some length with apprentices, those who are there to learn.

When Guillermo was 20 years old (he is now past 60) and was done with his bachelor's degree in pharmacology, he became interested in traditional medicine as well, since it seemed to him to work better than Western techniques in many cases. He decided to start an apprenticeship, which was very difficult at first, because "the spirits refused to communicate." Then he did it the hard way: he went to the rain forest alone for a year, with two pairs of pants, two shirts, a bow, three arrows, and a machete. He came back a shaman.

Guillermo still occasionally goes through a long diet of two months' duration. He states that continuing apprenticeship in this way throughout one's lifetime is a sign of a real curandero (as opposed to a charlatan). He taught healing to his son, James, who started working as a curandero in Pucallpa in 2007. James also learned a lot about plants from doña María, Guillermo's mother, who still participates in Guillermo's ceremonies and sings icaros.

An Interview with Guillermo Arrévalo

Guillermo Arrévalo is author of two books on botanical healing, and is a respected member of his indigenous community, the Shipibo-Conibo tribe. Also a critic of charlatan healers, he was interviewed by Rumrrill, in Spanish, in Pucallpa, Peru in November 2005. Arrévalo argued that drug tourists come to Peru to try to resolve personal problems in a form of self-encounter.

They try to liberate themselves from their problems or the psychological traumas that they suffer. By seeking a true spiritual path, many expect to cure a variety of physical illness. Arrévalo says that many of these people suffer from depression, or else are enslaved by their work. Others are materialistic and have neglected the spiritual part of themselves. Many of the tourists have been badly treated by their families, often particularly traumatized by their fathers' behavior toward them.

Interestingly, many of these tourists have taken other drugs and have traveled all over the world to obtain them. The Europeans frequently use LSD, hashish, and marijuana in elevated doses, which have resulted in negative experiences, psychosis, and psychological upheaval. Many tourists suffer from fear and paranoia. Arrévalo estimated that 80 percent of his female clients suffered rape trauma in their past. A large number are involved in a spiritual search. Arrévalo points to a steady increase in the number of patients of both sexes who come to the city of Pucallpa, Peru.

He argues that the tourist should know something about the person he has entrusted himself to in the drug session and should determine whether that person is truly knowledgeable. The client should verify the reputation of the individual practitioner with whom he deals. Arrévalo has commented on a large number of new shamans at work. In Pucallpa, many pretend they are healers—even among the indigenous Shipibo peoples. In San Francisco de Yarina Cocha, a Shipibo Indian community about one hour from Pucallpa, one finds shamans who gives tourists ayahuasca to drink—they are in almost every house. Arrévalo said that in the past, the curandero was a person of high social status within the community's hierarchy, with only one or two found in any community; this has changed dramatically and they have multiplied, not because of increased interest or a search for knowledge, but rather simply as a way to make money.

The number of apprentices to authentic shamans is fast diminishing. The reason is that the apprentice has to submit to a rigorous diet for a long period of time. Societal changes also affect this phenomenon. Young people want to live in cities and some go to the capital, Lima, to study. To become a healer, there are rules that have to be followed, and many young people are not disciplined enough to do so. Many Shipibo youth do not want to stay in their indigenous communities and to farm, fish, and hunt. The city is alluring to them. Many give up their cultural roots to fit into a mestizo identity. Some become involved in a variety of mysticism-linked activities, such as Rosicrucian texts, books of prayers and incantations, and occult sciences. Poverty is widespread in the city of Pucallpa, and the Shipibo, too, are mired in poverty. Let's look now at the actual text of the Rumrrill interview with Arrévalo.

INTERVIEW

An Interview with Roger Rumrrill and Guillermo Arrévalo, a Shipibo Urban Shaman[31]

RR: Tell me, what is the situation with shamanism at this point in time in the Amazon, particularly in Pucallpa, Peru?

GA: Well, regarding the theme of shamanism, there are two areas to discuss. One is folkloric shamanism, and the other is the practice, realization, and authenticity of the shaman.

RR: You're speaking first about folkloric shamanism, right? What is that about?

GA: I call it that because it deals with tourist attention, especially taking ayahuasca, with different ceremonial practices of singing that are conducted not only for healing. Traditional shamanism was for curing ceremonies. In the current situation, the shamans practice in Pucallpa and Iquitos. For me, this is merely folkloric.

RR: Is this folkloric shamanism that you refer to increasing because not only is it being practiced in Pucallpa and Iquitos, but there is also a growing tendency for shamanism to occur in other areas of the Amazon—in Brazil, Bolivia, and Ecuador? Do you think this folkloric shamanism is now in vogue?

GA: In my interpretation, most of all this is a type of commercial shamanism done in order to extract money from people. Many of those who are called shamans are not really shamans. Sure, they give ayahuasca to people to drink, but they don't do it like real shamans. Because of the business nature of their activity, they have to employ and promote this type of shamanism, and generally they do it throughout all the world. In Europe, there are persons who have learned to go around taking ayahuasca, but they don't have the force or energy that comes from the plant. Nor do the authorities pay attention to real shamans. Since it is a commercial undertaking, and since the community lives from tourism, for this reason, governmental authorities haven't considered that taking ayahuasca is not bringing benefits to the community. It can cause social-ecological consequences for some people who take the plant that I'll talk about shortly [Editor's note: Arrévalo is speaking in terms of family and community consequences].

RR: What stimulates the North Americans and Europeans in their search to experience Amazon shamanism? Why do these people come? What are they looking for? What is their objective? Their passion? You have seen many cases. Tell me, what do you think about this? What do they talk to you about?

GA: Principally, these tourists come to try to resolve personal problems. They say it is a self-encounter. They want to find the solution to their own problems and then to liberate themselves from those problems or the psychological traumas that they suffer. Others look for spiritual responses. They want to know the true spiritual path. They know other forms of what is a spiritual field. This is a more intellectual search for them. What is practiced by the Amazon shamans is a type of spirituality that is more complex, which distinguishes between the material and the spiritual. The other theme for Europeans and Americans is how to develop their spirit—the psyche of the person. Still others want to cure a variety of physical illnesses.

RR: Does this mean there is a spiritual crisis, and also a psychological one in the European and North American communities? This search for personal healing wasn't always so strong in the past. Today, those searching have increased considerably in number. Are Americans experiencing a spiritual crisis? Is that what you perceive in treating these patients?

GA: That's what I see. It is clear among many people. Indeed, many of them also suffer from depression. Others are enslaved by their work. Others are hooked into materialism and they have been neglectful of the spiritual part of themselves. Many of them have been badly treated by their family. They suffer emotionally from this, often from their fathers' behavior toward them. This happens both to Europeans and Americans—this depression.

RR: Have you recently seen any cases of loneliness and profound spiritual problems over the last few months?

GA: Yes, lately I've had patients who have used other drugs, all over the world. The Europeans use a lot of LSD, hashish, and marijuana. Many of them at times take elevated doses of these substances. They suffer a type of psychosis and psychological upheaval. They suffer from fear, paranoia, and other problems. These patients are ones that I treat with ayahuasca. Of course I had to develop my own consciousness to be able to help them psychologically. There are other cases where women have suffered from rape trauma, caused by a father, brother, or friend. These patients also suffer from depression, carrying those memories around for a long time and they don't accept their situation.

RR: Are there numerous cases of rapes, to indicate a tendency among your clients that shows these violations have increased in the United States and Europe? How many of your clients have suffered rape trauma?

GA: In my estimation, 80 percent among women. This causes me to think a lot about what goes on in developed countries. Here in Peru and in the Amazon one doesn't see so many of these upheavals. Also, I have seen spiritual losses. This is a very important theme. Among the cases I treated, 80 percent also were searching spiritually.

RR: How do you use ayahuasca to treat these difficult cases, these traumas that evidently originated in rapes, physical illness, obsession for money, or loneliness?

GA: First, what I do is to give the patient ayahuasca. Generally, these people want to have an ayahuasca experience. Since it produces a trance, I am prepared to develop my own consciousness to find the cause of their problem. I begin to work with them, the psychological part of the person, Mostly, I have to organize my work around what the person accepts as their beliefs about what it is that has damaged them, the particular trauma involved. On this basis, I organize the psychological part of the person, which enables me to understand and to see the solution to their problem. In this manner, the person can overcome his/her problem.

RR: If we think about European or American society having these problems, these crises, don't you think these potential patients will continue to increase in number? In the months and years to come, then, there could be a virtual invasion by clients who want to take ayahuasca, both Europeans and Americans, to try to cure themselves of their problems.

GA: Yes, we see this clearly in the steady increase in the number of patients.

RR: What is happening to human beings, from your point of view as a shaman, from your knowledge of human behavior in the twenty-first century? Where is humanity going?

GA: There are a large number of people who are turning to natural medicine. Various trends need to be looked at: there are some people who seek to transform natural resources and synthesize the plants. There are others who seek to use medicinal plants in their natural state. These two tendencies are followed by young people. What I believe is that it is important to preserve nature, because that is life. If the natural environment disappears, really, the earth will suffer a tremendous catastrophe. That's what I see.

RR: You say that it is laughable that the number of patients increases among Europeans and Americans searching for shamans in the Amazon. But, you have also shown that many of these supposed shamans are people without experience, people who are liars and cheats, people who don't have the capacity, the preparation, or the boldness to do this work. Many clients arrive in the Amazon and find themselves in the hands of these liars and traffickers.

GA: Yes, we see lot of that. Many who say they are healers don't know how to cure. In the case of someone who arrives with an illness such as rheumatism, or arthritis, these false shamans say such and such a plant is good for the particular illness. They give the prepared potion to the client, but get no results. The important thing is that the healer must know if the illness is really rheumatism or arthritis. If that is the case, there are really good plants available which are used for those types of illnesses. If these Europeans or Americans patients go to the liars, also they constrain the work of real healers.

RR: But, at the same time, this can cause problems, don't you think? If a patient has the intention to present himself to be cured, and the healer is a liar, then the outcome can become worse.

GA: Yes, there have been such cases. Some people arrive at my house, tricked that way. They have to be rescued, helped, so that this tourist doesn't take away with him or her a bad concept of the Amazon shaman.

RR: What about a serious case where a supposed shaman has tried to cure with plants not appropriate for the illness involved? The shaman may not know anything about healing. Could that cause madness or death? Has that happened?

GA: Yes, that can happen. In Pucallpa and other places, there have been people who have taken ayahuasca, but these potions were prepared with a number of additional plants. These other plants contain toxic substances. The tourist was not prepared for those plants which can have damaging effects. We see desperate cases where the patients have to go to the hospital. They need then to be given other pharmaceutical medicines. They may even die or go mad. Regarding madness, this depends on the shaman. It is up to him to be able to keep the patient from going crazy, if he can avoid those symptoms. A person who is not in control of these energies can cause grave consequences to the patient.

RR: How can we prevent European and American patients or those from other nationalities from falling into the hands of these liars and traffickers of traditional medicine? What should be done in that type of case? On the one hand, we have those cases that result in bad outcomes. This is a strategy for Amazon shamans. Then there is the danger that an individual will get worse after treatment and become mad. What do you think about this?

GA: What I think is that the tourist must know very well the person to whom he is entrusting himself for healing objectives. He should know all about the curandero and if that person is truly knowledgeable. He needs to verify the value of the individual practitioner with whom he deals.

RR: You speak about ayahuasca with toxic additives. Which ones are toxic?

GA: There are a number of different plants that are toxic, which many people are not prepared to handle, and there will be bad consequences. Also, if the tourist has taken other pills, even an antibiotic, yet another toxicity can poison him and even cause a cardiac arrest or other symptoms. Ayahuasca by itself is okay. It is prepared with chacruna or other plants that don't contain toxic elements. The toxic plants include toé, or datura. Since these are psychoactive plants which contain strong toxic elements, they can cause worse consequences, both toxicity and psychological problems. There are many people who use toé. These substances are toxic and dangerous. They can cause damage in the optic area and provoke blindness.

RR: Nowadays, looking at Pucallpa, how many of these tricksters, these false curanderos, would you estimate are at work? Are they few in number?

GA: There are a large number involved. Now in Pucallpa, there is a wave of competition that exists. Many here pretend that they are curanderos, even among indigenous people. In San Francisco de Yarina Cocha[Editor's note: This is a Shipibo Indian community about one hour's distance from Pucallpa], in almost every house there is a "shaman" or curandero. They give patients ayahuasca to drink.

RR: In the past among the Shipibo, the curandero or maestro was a person of high social status within the community's hierarchy. There might be only one or two in a community who were shamans, isn't that so? But that has multiplied, not because of a search for knowledge, but rather as a way to obtain money.

GA: Yes, it is for that reason. Moreover, it is dangerous.

RR: To begin this conversation, you spoke about two types of shamanism—the folkloric type, which we have just analyzed, and the other type—authentic shamanism. Tell me about this latter type of shamanism. How is ayahuasca used in that system which you called an authentic genre?

GA: In this field there are specialists, true practitioners, people who are knowledgeable about shamanism. For example, as some people have written, that there are those that have knowledge of plants and their magical management. At another level, there are "los mureyas," who have a deep knowledge regarding the administration of medicinal plants, as well as the magical aspects of nature. Then, there are those who can manage magical information—persons who can pass on to another level of knowledge, about the earth, the water, et cetera. They can transport themselves to other planes. Still other knowledge is called "bomanuna," which signifies persons who are surrounded by special states of consciousness. They can make bomanuna happen. They are developed people who at their level of consciousness can make things happen and they develop their sixth sense [Editor's note: This is called the "vidente phenomenon"].[32]

RR: Is that another level? We are now speaking now about two types of ayahuasca healers in a different hierarchy. One doesn't hear much about this "bomanuna." Is this from the Shipibo hierarchy or from other indigenous people?

GA: It is Shipibo-Conibo.

RR: Is the highest level the mureya? Or the bomanuna? How many mureyas are there in the Ucayali River region now?

GA: I think there could be three to four of these individuals.

RR: Are you one?

GA: Yes.

RR: Are these hierarchies very limited? Is the number of maestros expanding and growing? What is the situation nowadays?

GA: They are diminishing in number. The reason is that one has to submit to a diet that is very rigorous, a discipline, for over a long period of time. Thus, this diet causes consequences. Many times young people don't want to continue this type of apprenticeship. Actually, the majority of healers use ayahuasca, they smoke tobacco and utilize other inferior teaching plants, not the good ones. Before, if one wanted to be a shaman, one had to go on a diet for at least a year. Now, people don't want to try to arrive at such a high level.

RR: You speak about hierarchies among these maestros. The diet is an important factor in achieving power at the highest level. Given the situation of poverty that we see now in the Amazon, the population is very marginal, especially among indigenous peoples. Is this factor an obstacle for young people who want to learn to be apprentices to shamans? Is this the reason why the higher level of achievement doesn't happen any more?

GA: It is mostly because there are changes that have occurred in society today. Generally, young people want to live in cities. Some go to Lima to study. They have other goals. To function in this world of shamanism or "curanderismo" demands a certain measure of discipline, to live within the rules. Young indigenous people in these times don't want to get involved in these studies. They want to have a "normal" life. They prefer not to submit themselves to that type of strenuous apprenticeship.

RR: How much have the indigenous peoples of the Amazon changed, in this case, among the Shipibo, from your memory of your childhood to the present time? What have been the economic changes, the cultural changes, the changes in customs? These are major changes, irreversible ones, that have occurred in the Ucayali region. Do people continue to keep their ancient essential cultural values? Radical changes include the lessening of attachment to their cultural roots? How do you see this?

GA: We can say that there have been great changes over the last years, perhaps as much as a 60 percent change. Many Shipibo youth seek to change their customs. For example, they don't want to stay in their communities. In the past, they dedicated themselves to farming, fishing, and hunting, all those activities; generally, nowadays, young people go to the cities. Some expect to return home while others don't. Thus, some renounce their cultural roots. Also, many who are interested in shamanism don't want to submit themselves to diets with teaching plants. They prefer to have recourse to books of occult sciences. Others learn black magic, red magic, green magic, and white magic [Editor's note: These are different types of magic, such as love magic, magic for economic success, etc]. Also, they obtain information from other books of prayers and incantations, books about St. Cipriano, [Editor's note: Said to be the patron saint of curanderos], Rosicrucian texts, mysticism—there is an immense change. Indigenous youth seek other types of development. Economically speaking, it is the same—I can say that many indigenous people have worked in the lumber industry. But, in that field they didn't reach any great economic position. They obtained money for their work, but it was badly used. Nowadays, many don't have any money left from that period. Poverty is worse than before. I see that isn't a problem of a country, but rather a problem for the individual. If a person doesn't control or administer his earnings well, of course he will become part of a group of poor people. Even though the Shipibo have a lot of wealth in the elaboration of weavings, and artisanry, they also are mired in poverty due to a lack of awareness, a lack of development to find a better standard of living.

RR: This migration, the fleeing of young people to the cities like Pucallpa and Lima, is a process of change that...will fundamentally affect the identity and culture of the Shipibo. What do you think?

GA: Yes, this will have immense effects. Organically, the leadership doesn't know how to lead. False pride and egotism exist among the leaders.

RR: There are many changes that have occurred in the Amazon, from a political, cultural, educative, economic, and demographic approach. However, these have not been changes for the better. Everything appears to go backwards with regard to the economy. The changes in the Amazon over the last 30 years have worsened the economy. What values, if any, have remained from the Shipibo culture? Or has nothing remained?

GA: What has remained has been the knowledge base. For example, women still have knowledge of handicrafts, and there is knowledge of shamanism also, which can be used in economic development, if the Shipibo begin to value this. Shamanism is spiritual knowledge, which for the indigenous person can help himself overcome the economic recessions in which we are now living. This is an alternative.

RR: With regard to renewable resources of the Amazon: wood, soils, fish, et cetera, these are beginning to be scarce and to disappear. What remain in the Amazon as renewable resources?

GA: Knowledge is the renewable resource of the Amazon. If a people don't have knowledge, really, if it becomes lost, one will not know how to find the way to development in the future. If one doesn't have knowledge, one lives in a truly poor community.

RR: Indigenous peoples are a bank of knowledge which is visible. Where is that knowledge? That knowledge of the forests, of the rivers?

GA: Everything is there—the indigenous people have this knowledge.

RR: Everything has been sacked...

GA: But the knowledge still remains. I believe that no one has taken it away. Thus, we have to set off on the path of improvement on the basis of our knowledge. There is no other way to development.

*   *   *

Shipibo Belief Systems

A distinguished French anthropologist also trained in physical chemistry—Jacques Tournon[33]—has worked for many years with the Shipibo Indians of Pucallpa. He has delved into ayahuasca shamanism and achieved great rapport among the Shipibo Indians. Tournon has described some 17–20 different hallucinogenic plants, or additives to them, that healers use to cure. Some are quite toxic. The following discussion is based on his work with the Shipibo. The Shipibo believe that in their world of animism, not only do animals have a life force but birds, fish, places, and plants do as well. Also among the mestizo men and women studied by de Rios, in the 1960s and 1970s, ayahuasca and other plants were seen to be animated by a mother spirit—in the case of the ayahuasca vine, a boa constrictor. Some animals and plants, according to Tournon, are believed to have souls or spirits called *rao.* The Shipibo shamans use these spirits to heal. Some Shipibo shamans are called *meraya*—those who see. Shamans called the *onanya* invoke the spirits when they imbibe ayahuasca, which helps them to diagnose the client's illness. The Shipibo shamans' songs during the ayahuasca sessions are sung in a special voice, higher than the usual pitch. Historically, Catholic priests instituted Quechua, the language of the Inca, as a lingua franca throughout Peru. We still see this influence in areas without direct Inca influence, like in the Amazon. The songs that are sung are said to originate from the *rao yoshin,* the intrinsic spirit of the plant or animal. Both the healing shaman and the brujo, or witch, take over the spirits of the plants and enter into contact with them. A shaman does this in order to draw on the spirits' power, so he can diagnose and cure his client's illness.

There is a real difference among some individuals who simply use the rao plants. A special group who have access to an esoteric domain use these rao yoshin plants. The highly evolved shamans—either the onanya or meraya—had long periods of apprenticeship under the guidance of a specialist. The shaman drinks various rao drinks and follows special diets. Plants such as toé, *canachiari, chiricsanango,* and other decoctions are given to them by their teachers. Some of the specialists are not in an esoteric realm but have access to material knowledge of the healing plants—that is, knowledge open and accessible to all who are interested.

The Shipibo distinguish between the onanya, "those who know," and the meraya, "those who see." The meraya is more powerful than the onanya. Shape-shifting is a universal shamanic theme, where the shaman metamorphizes into the body of a powerful familiar; this was believed to be done by the meraya. The soul of the meraya leaves the body during the ayahuasca ceremony. The shaman has the power to transform himself into a spirit, showing his shamanic power par excellence. Merayas not only cure physical illness, but their realm of expertise includes treating behavioral issues and psychological problems of their clients. Both the onanya and the meraya are groups of shamans who have had long apprenticeships, during which time they encounter the spirits of the plants. The healer asks the spirits to teach him songs—icaros—and to provide him with knowledge. In this period of learning, the new shamans will develop powers of clairvoyance and gain esoteric knowledge. The apprentices receive patients and use the hallucinogenic plants to communicate with the *yoshin* spirits of other plants. Nineteenth century missionaries who observed these rituals believed that the devil himself or his demons were surely involved.

The actual diets of the apprentices consist of a few plantains and a little *chicha* (corn beer); they also must abstain from sex. During the healing ceremonies, which are quite public, the healer sucks out the thorn, or virote, said to be introduced into the client's body by a witch. These healers divine the future and resolve their client's personal problems.

The Bufeo (Dolphin)

In the Amazon, the *bufeo,* or sweet-water dolphin, is seen as a super predator. Unlike the Hollywood version of the friendly, bomb-diffusing creature, the dolphin is believed to have lots of power to seduce women, after it metamorphizes into human shape. Tournon tells us that bufeos are believed able to impregnate bathing women from a distance. Any children born from these unions are said to be white skinned. The dolphin lives under the water and has a life parallel to earth-bound humans. As a powerful spirit helper, he can teach the shaman the secrets of fishing. The shaman, when healing, calls on his spirits to dominate his adversaries. If he is able to do this, then he is able to heal his client's illness.

Every living being, whether animal or vegetal, as well as geographic sites, rivers, or hills, has a yoshin spirit. These spirits can be the etiological agents that cause illness. Rao is the term used for medicinal plants, some of which have powerful spiritual force as well. The onanya, who sees spirits, drinks brews made from hallucinogenic plants like ayahuasca. The onanya sees the yoshin rao and invokes them to come to see the patient and diagnose the illness. This can either be a natural illness or one provoked by a witch. During the ayahuasca session, the onanya sings in languages not known to his fellows, like Quechua and Piro (another Indian language). The songs come from the rao yoshin, and they are lent to the healers. The yoshin is the intrinsic spirit of the plant or animal. The *ibo* is flesh and bones—a person or an animal—and includes the mother spirit of the plant or animal. As mentioned earlier, in urban settings, the mother spirit of the ayahuasca plant is said to be the boa constrictor, widely admired as a hunter due to its ability to move quietly and effortlessly through the jungle.

During ayahuasca sessions, the shaman or the witch enters into contact with the spirit of the plants. The intrinsic powers of the plants permit the healers to diagnose and cure. This is part of an esoteric realm not readily available to the casual observer. Regarding the material use of the rao plants, the shamans who are accomplished in their skills (or highly evolved), the ona-nya or meraya, follow an apprenticeship period and participate in numerous sessions as assistants. They drink various plant decoctions and follow various diets. They learn to take toé and chiricsanango, both powerful hallucinogens, and they also take decoctions or cuttings of trees in cane alcohol, which contain powerful chemicals, hallucinogens in their own right. They learn diverse melodies to distinguish the spirits of the plants, the earth, and water, as well as to diagnose illnesses. They take care of patients and use hallucinogenic plants that permit them to communicate with the yoshin spirits.

Since the nineteenth century, diverse missionaries have commented on these pagan specialists from the perspective of their own world view. They labeled these shamans as devils or demons. Today in anthropological hind-sight, we would better translate these as spirits. Historical accounts tell about shamans who smoked a large cigar and then sucked out the thorn (virote) that was said to have been introduced into the patient's body by a witch to cause the patient illness. As the result of the ayahuasca healers' special diets, they were weakened from taking in little food. They were also forbidden to have sex with their wives. During the healing ceremonies, they sucked at the afflicted area of the patient's body and removed a thorn so that the client's health would return. De Rios described one such ceremony performed by an itinerant healer in Iquitos in 1968, when dozens of people flocked into a thatched house at the river's edge to see the healer suck out an ugly black substance, which was said to be the virote. This was introduced by a witch. Only then could the elderly female patient be cured. One could have heard a pin drop in the thatched house, given the rapt attention of the observers that the healer controlled in the moment of healing.

José Curitima Sangama of the Cocama–Cocamilla Tribe: Shoals of Achual Tipishca in the Peruvian Amazon

The Cocama-Cocamilla of Peru are the descendants of the thousands of Tupi Guarani, who for more than 4,000 years occupied the Amazon basin from the delta of the Marajó River to the mouth of the Amazon River, which empties into the Atlantic Ocean. They built a pre-Colombian civilization and established themselves at the basin of the Huallaga River in Peru for about a thousand years. Then, as the result of a large and bloody dispute with the Pano Indians for hegemony of the area around the rich basin of the Ucayali River,[34] along with other accomplishments, the indigenous group became known to have the best curanderos in the lower Amazon. For perhaps more than 100 years, they were established in the lagoon of Achual Tipishca, an offshoot of the lower Huallaga River, a town where their center of Amazonic shamanism achieved renown.

José Curitima Sangama was born in Achual Tipishca and is recognized today as one of the most adept curanderos of the Cocama-Cocamilla tribe. The interview to follow, conducted by Rumrrill, took place on November 12, 2006, and registers the dynamic of the changes and transformations that operate in all aspects of Amazonian life and culture.

Don José is 70 years old and has been curing since the age of 20. In Achual Tipishca, he went through his apprenticeship and learned from other "grand masters" of curanderismo; his only son is currently studying to become a Catholic priest. He says that the icaros (mariris) are the most important part of the healing. They are designed to combat a specific disease or reinforce the healing activity of a particular plant. Also, he may invoke animals to strengthen the patient (a jaguar is called upon against general weakness; a vulture, against digestive illnesses, because a vulture can eat everything, and so on).

He does not pay attention to dosages or appear to know about any contraindications of the ayahuasca tea. During the ceremony, he drinks aguardiente right before taking ayahuasca. He accepts all tourists, of which there are only a few in Lagunas. He claims that other curanderos in Achual Tipishca "are afraid of these gringos," which is perhaps the reason why don José moved to Lagunas. Recently he gave ayahuasca tea to two tourists. In his opinion, the ayahuasca drink, once prepared with the correct amounts of ayahuasca and chacruna, is not dangerous to take, because he has already blown tobacco smoke over the drink and chanted mariris while preparing it, thus magically protecting the clients. In his perception, no harm could come to any of his clients.

He laments that there are lots of charlatans in Lagunas, who take 500–600 soles (up to $200) for a ceremony, while he usually asks for about 50 soles (about $16). He blames his poor living situation on the jealousy of charlatans, who somehow attract all potential clients. Don José cures daño, "choque del aire," "pulsario," and other culture-specific diseases that are mostly psychosomatic. In one treatment session, don José did not use any plants but conducted the ceremony with only a little amount of *timolina* sprayed on the patient's head.

Don José believes that, in general, he works with the help of God, who after all created all the plants. However, he does not chant mariris to ask for God's protection. Instead, he directly contacts plant spirits during the ceremony, although he is influenced by Roman Catholic ritual and called upon "La Virgen de Dolores" in one of his icaros. In addition to plant spirits, he invokes the spirits of tobacco, water, earth, and space. He believes that stars are especially helpful against fever. He invites the beings that live "above the sky, on the ice." These look like little gray men, and, guided by don José, can cure high fever, since in his opinion, they obviously never get hot.

INTERVIEW

An Interview with the Indigenous Shaman José Curitima Sangama

RR: Achual Tipishca, in the lower Huallaga River, is like the capital of Amazonic shamanism. I remember having walked through the town, through some of the few streets there, and I had the sensation that everyone who walked through the town was a shaman. How many curanderos or shamans are there in this territory? Or, perhaps, are they disappearing as in other areas of the Amazon?

JCS: The shamans didn't disappear. Now there are only four left: Jorge Caritimari, Miguel Manihuari, and myself. The other one I have forgotten right now his name. But there are four of us who are left healing.

RR: In one of my trips to Achual Tipishca, I observed the cultural changes that we can see in all the Amazon. One of these changes refers to shamanism. I was told that in Achual Tipishca, the curanderos no longer used ayahuasca in their rituals and cures, but only tobacco. All of them have became tobacco healers. When I asked why the curanderos were now tobacco healers, they told me that ayahuasca was no longer available. With the deforestation of the jungle by people who want to build farms and extract wood, ayahuasca also has disappeared. Do these practicing shamans of Achual Tipishca use tobacco or ayahuasca?

JCS: They continue to use ayahuasca because it is a medicinal plant that accompanies us in our healing and serves us to make good medicines. For this reason we continue to use ayahuasca, but we also use tobacco.

RR: Isn't it true that in shamanism, there are hierarchies and levels of achievement? In mestizo life, the highest level is "el banco." In the Shipibo-Conibo Indians, the highest level is "meraya." Among the Ashaninka it is the "shiripiari." Among Andean shamans who speak Quechua, the highest level is the "alto mesayoc," and among the Aymara Indians, it is the "yatiri." Among the Cocama-Cocamilla of Achual Tipishca, what is the highest level called?

JCS: Among the Cocama-Cocamilla we also call that level "banco."

RR: Are you a banco?

JCS: I am a banco.

RR: Because a banco, the same as a meraya, flies like a bird and travels under the water like a fish. Can you do that?

JCS: I work under the water like a dolphin. There I concentrate on my healing.

RR: I remember that there were times in which you went to the hills, to the center, as you call it, to undergo a special diet. Do you continue going to the mountain to diet?

JCS: I continue to diet. I go to the hills to diet with special foods.

RR: During that time, I suppose you have no woman with you.

JCS: I also include no women in my diet.

RR: During the last several years shamanism was seen as a universal style in the world. Tourists from Europe and the United States come to take ayahuasca. They come to the Amazon to cure their physical illnesses, but more come because of spiritual reasons. These travelers almost always prefer to work with indigenous shamans. Have you received any of these "gringos"?

JCS: They always come. And I have cured many. They also come to record the songs, the mariris, and to see how we cure patients. All the gringos are interested in this.

RR: Have you treated some of them lately? Where do they come from?

JCS: Yes, recently I treated one man from the United States. He liked the music I used very much and the form of my work. We went to the forest area to take the special diet.

RR: What illnesses were you treating and curing?

JCS: I cure mal aire, saladera [Editor's note: Negative energy of people, and misfortune illness], as well as other sicknesses. To do the healing, I ask people to come to my house and in my house and remain there for a while. I take their pulse to know what illness they have. According to the illness that the patient has causes me to determine if I will use tobacco or ayahuasca.

RR: When do you use tobacco and when do you use ayahuasca?

JCS: It depends on the illness. If the illness isn't a serious one, I use timolina. [Editor's note: The herb thyme.] If the illness is serious, I use tobacco so I can solve the patient's problem. I use ayahuasca to better understand the patient's illness. It is how the doctors in hospital do it, like a diagnosis.

RR: Who cures? Is it the curandero or the mother of the plant, the "ayahuascamama"?

JCS: It's the mother of the plant that cures. She tells us which song to sing, and which music we should use to cure the patient. We accompany the mother of the plant.

RR: People say that each day there is less and less ayahuasca in the Amazon, and above all, in the Huallaga basin. Is that true?

JCS: There is ayahuasca. Many people are planting it. I also plant it and my ayahuasca is growing very nicely. An engineer came the other day from Yurimaguas and asked us to grow ayahuasca, because he says that it will go for a good price. People from all over are going to be looking for ayahuasca.

RR: Where did you plant ayahuasca? Was it in the town of Achual Tipishca, or in the forest, far from the town?

JCS: My ayahuasca is in the hills. Ayahuasca has a secret. It has to be alone in order for it to grow and twine up nicely. The secret is in that it shouldn't be seen by women, especially any women who have their menstrual period or who have not slept well, due to drunkeness, et cetera. If those women see the ayahuasca, the plant becomes resentful and neither grows nor twines upright. It folds over and is damaged. On the other hand, when ayahuasca is alone, it grows nicely, and when you are intoxicated with it, it's good and normal.

RR: I remember one night that I took ayahuasca with you in Lagunas. After a moment in the middle of the intoxication, you invoked and called out to a shaman who had died a long time ago. He began to speak through your mouth. I was astonished to listen to this thickened voice of someone who had died about 100 years ago and who spoke through your mouth. Who was it?

JCS: I don't remember who it was. Some years have passed since then.

RR: But you continue making these invocations and entreaties to shamans who have died, and you ask that they come and help you in the healing ceremonies, don't you?

JCS: I continue to call on them. Because this is the principal basis of healing. They are my teachers who show me how to heal. For that reason, I call them and they come and teach me the music. With that, I am able to cure.

RR: At what age did you begin to cure?

JCS: I began to cure at age 20, thanks to the teachings that my father gave me. He was a good plant healer (a "vegetalista"). When he died, I took over his work in town and the care of his patients.

RR: When you die, who will replace you?

JCS: I don't know. Perhaps someone who shows an interest. I have only one son.

RR: Perhaps you'll have other children. Can you still have children?

JCS: I can, but my wife can't any longer. As they say in Achual Tipishca, her resin is all dried up.

RR: How old is your wife?

JCS: She is 52 years old—with dried resin.

RR: Returning to the theme—the gringos who come to Achual Tipishca, what are they looking for?

JCS: They come to take ayahuasca, to look at and to study the plants, the animals, and to see how the life of people is here.

RR: A short time ago, a journalist from the United States came here to report on shamanism. I told him about you and how to find you. Did he come?

JCS: I didn't meet him because now I live in Lagunas. I moved there so that my son could study at school.

RR: Once I saw in Lagunas a Cocama-Cocamilla who was huge. Taller than the gringos. Do you remember his name?

JCS: He is Venancio. He is also a healer. At times, he manages to heal well, at times, no.

RR: Among the Cocamilla youth, do they have any interest to learn about shamanism?

JCS: Very little. Almost no interest at all. On the other hand, before, when I was a boy, there was much interest, and our parents taught us. Now the youth don't want to take ayahuasca, nor smoke tobacco. They only smoke fine red store-bought packs of tobacco and when they see us smoke black tobacco, they make fun of us saying that that is for dirty witches.

RR: You haven't traveled much through the Amazon, at least physically. From Achual Tipishca you've gone to Lagunas and from Lagunas to Achual Tipishca. But surely you have heard people talk about the Amazon shamans, the healers among the Shipibo, Cocama-Cocamilla, Ashaninka, Yagua, Aguaruna, and other indigenous settlements in the Amazon. Which are said to be the best?

JCS: The best are the Cocama-Cocamilla. I have verified all. I'm not saying this because that's my tribe. No one can sing the icaros as well as the Cocama-Cocamilla.

RR: And why are they the best?

JCS: Because we know which illness the patient has. We pulse them and rapidly we know which illness they suffer. The others, in contrast, have to take their huayuza [Editor's note: An unspecified hallucinogen] in order to know what the illness is.

RR: But I knew a shaman, don Manuel Cordova-Rios, who didn't even need to pulse a patient. He only looked at the patient with his eyes and saw the interior of his body. Do you believe that is possible?

JCS: It's possible. I also look at patients and see into their interior. But now that my vision is bad, and I suffer from cataracts, I have to pulse the client and try to figure out what problem he has. The music is engraved in my mind and with that I can cure.

RR: Can we listen to some mariris? [Editor's note: Healing songs, called icaros in other parts of the Amazon.]

JCS: Which music do you want? To get women, to be successful in business, or to travel?

RR: For journeys. Tomorrow I leave on a trip.

JCS: Good, my friend Roger, I am going to make you dream about a music so that God can accompany you in your trip and nothing bad will happen to you. [He sings mariris.]

RR: In what language are you singing?

JCS: In Cocama-Cocamilla.

RR: I remember that in one shamanic session with you, there was someone who suffered from a stomach ailment. You sang the mariri, asked for the strength of the stomach of a vulture, and you said: "give his stomach the strength of a vulture who eats rotten meat and never suffers from stomach problems." For another patient who seemed thin and weak, you asked for the strength of an anteater. Do you invoke the strength of animals to heal your patients?

JCS: Yes, that's how it is. For a weak patient, we invoke a stone. The stone gives him the strength of a healthy man's body. For a weakness of the stomach, we call the spirit of the white vulture, of the pig, and other animals who eat rotten things and never suffer from nausea or stomach problems. We call upon serpents, ants, the odorous ant, the iguana, or butterfly, according to the illness.

RR: When a patient suffers from love problems, if a boyfriend or a wife has abandoned your client, which animal do you invoke to help them?

JCS: That's different. Because in the earlier cases, we were using the icaros for sick people. For love issues, we invoke the girl or person herself. You give me her full name and I call the girl by her name. I don't need her photo like other curanderos do. I utilize also a doll or a little altar on which I place the doll. Also, I use the huacanqui plant to give a fragrance to the body. We use also the leaf of a bijauito, very fragrant, and sangapilla. And if the girl doesn't love you, the black boa lends us its colors, and we adorn the face of the doll with the colors of the black boa. We also lend the doll its tongue. These are the secrets of love magic.

This discussion of Shipibo and Cocama native ayahuasca use, along with the Venezuelan Piaroa use of ayahuasca, contrasts dramatically with the drug tourism in the Amazon that we will look at in Chapter 3.

*   *   *

Two other native Cocama healers were interviewed. They use traditional techniques but have been influenced by forces of modernity, even in the isolated areas in which they live.

Don Javier is a mestizo, although his mother originated from a Cocama Indian tribe. He is 40 years old and has been healing for 20 years. He claims to have learned from his parents. He is said to be one of the most respected healers in the Achual Tipishca village. Currently, most curanderos have moved to a small town called Lagunas, or they have died without leaving apprentices to take over their work. Community members generally prefer pharmaceutical medications rather than plant remedies. Don Javier claims to cure fever, headaches, "body ache," and all kinds of daños (witchcraft hexes). He has very few patients. When he was asked to specify his methods, and to name a few plants for the most commonplace disorders, he was unable or perhaps unwilling to give a sufficiently clear reply. He holds ayahuasca ceremonies periodically and was quick to invite us to one. He did not appear however to be very credible, especially since he does not pay any attention to dosage variations or contraindications of the ayahuasca.

Don Javier believes in different kinds of magic which roughly correspond to the particular variety of ayahuasca he offers his clients during the ceremony: each variety of a different color—such as white, yellow, red, green, and black—corresponds to particular types of magic and witchcraft-caused illnesses. He spoke about how his body is possessed by a plant spirit or a jungle spirit as a natural part of the ceremony. It seems that this belief is found widely among Cocama curanderos in general. The healer is religious, but he does not work by directly calling on God, Jesus, or the saints to help in healing.

Don Felipe, an Indigenous Healer from Achual Tipishca

This healer is a 60-year-old Cocama Indian who has been working as a healer since his twenties. He learned from other curanderos in the Achual Tipishca area, where he used to work as well. A few years ago he moved out of the village to the Huallaga River area, about an hour away by canoe. He cures with plants and is an ayahuasquero and a *tabaquero* (he uses tobacco juice in some ceremonies, not only cigars). Don Felipe is extremely poor and lives in a jungle house (*tambo*) that does not have any walls, just thatched roofing . Both he and don José Curitima Sangama appear to have worse living conditions than many of their patients.

Icaros are the most important component in don Felipe's ayahuasca ceremonies. These incantations guide the spirits and allow the plants to work on the patient. Besides, only with icaros is it possible to call upon the spirit of some dead maestro, a curandero, and control that spirit for healing. He also believes that he is not responsible personally for curing. Rather, all the healing work is done by the spirit curanderos who come to possess don

Felipe's body during the ceremony. The healer is very reluctant to reveal more information about specific diseases, cures, plants, and so on, because he claims that "it's a secret." In our interviews we found that many of the shamans are quite willing to share their knowledge, to validate their work. Don Felipe does not pay attention to dosage levels for his clients or any contraindications of the ayahuasca tea. In don Felipe's ceremonies, participants often take ayahuasca to watch over their family members who are far away, or even dead. He does not believe that different types of ayahuasca exist or that they cause different visionary responses.

Modernization and its Effects on the Cocama–Cocamilla of Peru

The social, economic, cultural, and environmental changes in the Peruvian Amazon in the last decades are drastic and profound. As the population has increased, poverty, malnutrition, and the erosion of natural ecosystems have all occurred, especially with the flora and fauna of the region.

The indigenous community of the Cocama-Cocamilla is an example. Ten years ago, the community was located in the mouth of their lagoon on the Huallaga River. This was the center of Amazonic shamanism, as the Cocama-Cocamilla were reputed to be the wisest healers and shamans of the area, with a thousand-year-old tradition. Descended from the Tupi Guarani Indians, the Cocama-Cocamilla were one of the most ancient pre-Colombian civilizations found in the Amazon basin for at least 4,000 years.[35]

Ten years ago, José Curitima Caritimari and don Felipe were not the only masters of shamanism who lived in Achual Tipishca. There were at least a dozen more who cured the mestizo and white populations of Yurimaguas, the principal city of the lower Huallaga region and the capital of the province of Loreto, as well as in other nearby towns. At that time, there was less poverty and malnutrition, and many species of fish were found in the river and lagoons. In the space of 10 years, Achual Tipishca has tripled its population, with a poverty and malnutrition rate that is high. The rich lagoons of the past no longer exist. The indigenous fishermen, for whom the lagoon was the principal source of nutrition and protein, no longer have fish resources such as *paiche, gamitana, paco,* and other fish species of the region available to them. Along with the pauperization of the population, the lagoon has also dried up. And from the more than 20 healers of 10 years ago, only two or three young apprentices are left. The rest have died or migrated to the city of Yurimaguas, or to other nearby towns. Or, like José Curitima, who has moved to the town of Lagunas, many want their children to study in the secondary school. The axis mundi, the center of Amazonic shamanism, no longer exists. The case of Achual Tipishca reveals and expresses the great dynamic of changes that is encapsulating the Amazon. The indigenous populations are suffering dramatic modifications in their ability to survive, and shamanism, one of the most valiant expressions of the indigenous Amazonic culture, is suffering modifications and distortions.

One of the expressions of these changes is shamanic tourism, the mercantilization of traditional healing. In the next chapter we will look in great detail at drug tourism. Most ayahuasca healing today offered by indigenous tribal shamans or mestizo healers takes place in cities, at hotels run by tourist companies. In this zone, and others like it, authentic curanderos, mostly indigenous men, are very poor. Why are they generally poor? Perhaps because their knowledge and wisdom are not commercial. Rather, this knowledge is basically to serve other poor people, to heal them of their illnesses, historically for low fees. In this remote area of Peru, there is not much contact with foreigners seeking ayahuasca, or any real cash income for shamanic healing.

The town where José Curitima now lives, Lagunas, has a population of between 10,000–15,000 inhabitants. Perhaps 95 percent are indigenous Cocama-Cocamilla, It is the largest tribal city in the Amazon. However, Curitima is a marginal man due to the influence of urban culture. There is television, the internet, radio, and music, as well as the lifestyle and customs that come from big cities like Lima, Tarapoto, Iquitos, and Yurimaguas. This has relegated the expressions of the indigenous culture—shamanism—to the lowest social and cultural value in a society that has practically renounced its indigenous identity.

*   *   *

As we turn to a discussion of drug tourism, we need to keep in mind how social change is destroying the indigenous ayahuasca traditions at their most pristine level. These indigenous healers, with a few exceptions discussed earlier within the Shipibo or Cocama-Cocamilla tradition, have not become incorporated into the commercialization. This has become a runaway, free-for-all attempt to profit from ancient traditions by marketing and selling mystical experiences to foreigners.

CHAPTER 3

DRUG TOURISM

In 1994 de Rios first wrote about drug tourism[1]—where charlatans take individuals from the first world on tours to the Peruvian, Ecuadorian, and Brazilian Amazon to participate in plant hallucinogenic sessions with ayahuasca (various *Banisteriopsis* species). This tourism has increased over the years, due to lower travel costs and as the result of information freely and cheaply disseminated across nations. A single, unified global market has been created, despite the fact that additives to the ayahuasca tea are Schedule I drugs with heavy penalties in the United States. These plants contain the powerful chemicals harmine, harmaline, and tetrohydroharmaline. This phenomenon—a dark side of globalization—has increased in the last 15 years, causing serious health hazards for the clients of these "new-shamans." The giving of powerful psychedelics to a naïve audience by individuals without knowledge or training is potentially very dangerous, from a public health perspective. Unfortunately these problems have been poorly documented. These pseudo-healers were first discussed in 1974 by Carlos Alberto Seguin.[2] They are not unknown in South American healing traditions; urban middle-class men and women have, on occasion, usurped the traditional role of folk healer or curandero and thus contributed to the ongoing demise of the traditional cultural healing system.

A number of upscale, well-to-do, prominent Americans and Europeans are touring Amazonian cities. Interested neither in parrots nor piranhas, they revel in special all-night religious ceremonies presided over by a powerful shaman, and they drink a foul-smelling brew—the woody vine ayahuasca. Unlike the jungle denizens who for the last several thousand years have drunk the potion to see the vine's mother spirit—a boa constrictor—in order to protect themselves from enemies, to divine the future, or to heal their emotional and physical disorders, the urban tourist is on a never-ending search for self-actualization and growth. In this postmodern period where people no longer produce their own food, where the family has broken down, where there is a significant absence of community tradition and shared meanings, individuals are wracked with feelings of low self-esteem and confusion about values. They are compelled to fill the emptiness with the experience of receiving something from the world. Why not a mystical experience with divinity? From their travels they bring home outrageous stories, of the fabulous witch doctor encountered, of the vomiting and diarrhea, of the fast-moving kaleidoscopic visions, of the sounds and the smells of the jungle—wow! What a trip.

Unscrupulous practitioners who exploit the tourists abound, and they are conscious of the farce they perpetrate. In Amazonian cities, middle-class men become instant traditional healers without undergoing an apprenticeship period, without any teachers, and without any protective controls. They give tourists mixtures of 12 or more different psychedelic plants to help them mystically become embedded in the universe. Many are witchcraft plants that affect neurotransmitters, upset the balance of certain brain chemicals, and may even make it impossible to read or write for an entire year. These so-called shamans fight among themselves, and all have their champions abroad who function as travel agents and tour guides. A few make money, seduce women, and obtain personal power and control over others. Agents abroad often earn as much as $8,000 to $10,000 from a two-week trip.

Drug tourism is part of the phenomenon of international mass tourism, where millions of temporary travelers from industrialized nations seek in the margins of the third world a figment of their imagination, a fantasy of Western consciousness—the exotic, erotic primitive, or happy savage. The drug dilettantism has a special rhetoric, and travel literature includes terms like "advanced shamanic training." Expensive brochures printed on fine paper, costing thousands of dollars, boast of spiritual transformation techniques of jungle shamans. The Amazon is said to be the last remaining spiritual sanctuary on earth. By paying the cost of the trip, one becomes an impeccable warrior in the tradition of the writer Carlos Castaneda.

The phenomenon has become so flagrant since the mid-1980s that the culture of native peoples is in danger of extinction. New Age magazines invite readers to take guided tours to remote villages or sacred places of power. This is a deadly, contemporary weapon that hastens the demise of native cultures, as international drug enforcement treats this type of tourism as one more illegal activity and in some areas of the world persecutes native peoples involved with the tourists.

These tourists to the Amazon see exotic people of color untouched by civilization, close to nature. They do not see the civilizing influences in these areas of Catholic and Protestant missionary activity. Little do they know that the Amazonian city dwellers get better television reception than those who live in southern California, because of the major telecommunications satellites on the outskirts of their cities.

There is little hope for dialogue between the drug tourists and the Amazonians, whose traditions of ayahuasca use are linked in a matrix dealing with the moral order, with good and evil, with animals and humans, and with health and illness—this has little to do with the experiences and needs of people in industrial societies. There is an evil, exploitive aspect of this eco-touristic enterprise. Many of these so-called native healers are common drug dealers, dressed for deception. They provide the exotic setting and prep the tourist to have an "authentic personal experience." The drug tourism often leaves psychotic depression and confusion in its wake.

Modernization and cultural change over the last century have destroyed the material base of many Amazonian traditional cultures. Commercial shamanism in Peru has become a system, where foreigners are given a powerful plant psychedelic at a cost of $1,000–$1,500 per week during a visit, compared to the $20–$30 cost for local people. Since these drug rituals have become a commercial undertaking, and since the community lives from tourism, governmental authorities have not curtailed this activity, despite international treaties concerning drug interdiction. One of the additives to ayahuasca mentioned earlier, called chacruna in Peru (*Psychotropia viridis*), contains DMT. DMT is a prohibited Schedule I drug covered by the Controlled Substances Act of 1970.

We should examine the use of hallucinogenic plants by American and European tourists in Latin America. In particular, it is important to point out the role that anthropological scholars inadvertently have played as they have studied and analyzed traditional psychedelic rituals, despite the fact that they published in journals reviewed by their peers and in academic settings. Little does it matter that they presented their talks at academic conferences, or avoided sensationalizing their studies. In spite of this measured approach, the work of these scholars on esoteric rituals linked to drug ingestion has diffused to what has been called the "democratic masses," discussed in 1932 by the Spanish philosopher Ortega y Gasset.[3] There is a real difference between the new religions' sacramental use of plant hallucinogens—for example, that of the União do Vegetal Church (UDV) in Brazil,[4] to be discussed in Chapter 5—compared with trendy hallucinogenic ingestion by urban-educated baby boomers and New Age men and women. This drug tourism causes harm to participants. It also changes and effectively destroys traditional urban and rural hallucinogenic healing that has roots in the prehistoric past.[5]

In the process of examining esoteric drug rituals, the anthropologist and other social scientists must take responsibility, at some level, for the outcome of their work. There has been an increase in drug-related tourism, caused by unsuspecting men and women who are seeking help for their psychological problems, to alleviate past traumas, or who are looking for spiritual insights. However, before we rush to condemn the unsuspecting or uncaring tourist, we need to comprehend the charlatans in whose hands the tourists find themselves. These so-called "neo-shamans" are mostly men without any special training, with little—if any—knowledge of disease process or biochemistry, and who are prone to use local witchcraft plants (read *poisons*) to ensure that their clients have a good trip. Many of the plants used are quite toxic and cause damage to individuals. A number of the plants interact negatively with antidepressant medicines, as well as with antibiotics and common foods. Moreover, the suggestibility properties of these substances, first discussed by de Rios and Grob,[6] are, on occasion, used by some new ayahuasqueros to aid in the seduction of female participants in rituals.

Nightshade plants (the *solanaceae*) are dangerous to fool with. Even within the same plant, the alkaloid content can vary tremendously. Those collecting and preparing these plants often have no understanding of these factors, and illnesses and even fatalities can occur. Excessive doses lead to death through respiratory failure or cardiovascular collapse. Dosage is everything.

Drug Tourism: Merchandise and Commodity

A phenomenon that has been going on for several decades—drug tourism in the Amazon—includes the merchandising and commercialization of spiritual states of consciousness induced by drinking an admixture of several psychedelic plants. These plants have a long history of use by urban and rural mestizo healers, and by river-edge farmers and native groups. This tourism, with all the pageantry of a Hollywood epic film, is replete with tour guides and celebrity neo-shamans and charlatans. They are out to get rich quick. This situation is a public health menace and needs to be evaluated and controlled. This drug tourism is different from the sacramental use of these plants in new religions such as the União do Vegetal and Santo Daime in Brazil. Rather, this is materialistic exploitation of foreign visitors to the Amazon regions of South America, which makes a mockery of, and is destroying, the traditional use of such plants.

Media covered this topic of ayahuasca's sacramental use nationwide during the summer of 2006. The U.S. Supreme Court ruled on ayahuasca use within a branch of the UDV in Santa Fe, New Mexico, where 30 kilograms of the tea had been confiscated. An article on ayahuasca was featured in the Sunday,

January 6, 2006 *New York Times*. The ruling by the top U.S. court to allow ayahuasca use for religious purposes is relatively novel and still controversial.

Brief Description

One country's sacrament can be another country's illicit drug, as officials in South America and the United States are well aware. For centuries, the hallucinogenic tea made from a vine native to the Amazonian rain forest has been taken as a religious sacrament by members of several cultures in South America. Many spiritual leaders, shamans, and their followers consider the tea and its main components—ayahuasca and *Psychotropia viridis* (containing DMT)—to be both enlightening and healing. In fact, ayahuasca loosely translated means "vine of the spirit"—ayahuascamama. The sacrament has lured American and European visitors to South America to partake. These "drug tourists" are being put at risk by charlatans who are not actually shamans or religious figures, just profiteers. In the meantime, the ayahuasca vine has been at the heart of legal battles stemming in the United States, pulling in the U.S. Supreme Court. Some U.S. church groups are using ayahuasca in their ceremonies and have been fighting for government approval to do so. The União do Vegetal filed suit against the Drug Enforcement Administration after its U.S. leader was arrested in 1999, and 30 kilograms of the tea seized. The case culminated on February 21, 2006, when the Supreme Court ruled unanimously in favor of the UDV and its members' use of the tea. Opponents continue to fight its use, even as U.S. scientists and psychologists investigate whether ayahuasca has healing properties that might be put to conventional use for physical or mental health purposes.

The neo-shamans are generally charlatans who seek profits from their clients' trendy introduction to altered states of consciousness. Esoteric beliefs and experiences are available to the consumer for a high price and are supposedly derived from traditional urban healing or indigenous use patterns. With the help of the Peruvian journalist and writer Roger Rumrrill, interviews with 27 shamans were conducted. Two indigenous healers in Chapter 2 commented at length on the drug tourism they observe even in their remote locations, where psychologically troubled men and women come to seek help for depression and other ailments.

The New Shamans

The new shamans are basically businessmen who extract cash from visitors. Some of them develop foolish rituals and procedures that are burlesque images of what they believe an altered state should be. Some healers use mud baths and nudity in their group rituals, quite distinctive from traditional ayahuasca rituals that de Rios observed in 1968–1969, 1977, and 1979. Then, a simple plastic cloth was laid on the ground, and clients were seated around a circle with the healer whistling incantations (icaros) to provoke spiritual contact for a couple of hours.

Today drug tourists are not screened. New healers generally have not been apprenticed, nor have they fasted or adhered to special diets of the past. Predominantly mestizo middle-class men, with some women also involved, these new healers in many ways usurp the tradition of folk healers or curanderos, and thus they contribute to the ongoing demise of a cultural healing and religious system. Historically, ayahuasca was used to determine the source of witchcraft hexes and evildoing, and to permit a powerful shamanic healer to rectify his client's anxiety and fears and cause retribution of evil to the perpetrator.

The New Age Movement and Ayahuasca Tourists

In an important book, Paul Heelas[7] presents a profile of the New Age baby boomer and the world view that characterizes the dozens of drug tourists that the authors have interviewed over the last 20 years, in English, Spanish, and French. They emanate from the United States, Canada, and Europe. Heelas has clarified the major thrust of the values and views of these visitors. We can see how such New Age baby boomers would be attracted to ayahuasca rituals abroad. This contrasts dramatically with Peruvian patients who came to ayahuasca healers like don Hilde. Unlike a spirituality based on traditional religions of Christianity or Islam, for example, primary among drug tourists is the concept of self-spirituality. To the baby boomer seeking an ayahuasca experience, spirituality is believed to lie within the individual himself. One must find one's authentic nature and transform oneself. Implicit or explicit is the belief that society has conditioned or brainwashed the person. These individuals who come have profound dissatisfaction with mainstream values and identities. They believe that a powerful psychedelic like ayahuasca and an arduous trip to the Amazon will enable them to enter the realm of the "self." The hallucinogen will permit the individual to develop a special inner sensation or mood. Heelas estimates that there are more than 10 million individuals—a significant percentage of the U.S. population—who fit into this category. There is a quiet revolution going on with a strong middle and upper-middle class of professionals—these people are called "expressivists" in the language of sociology. They show a growing interest in pagan-type religions. Ayahuasca shamanism is a hot topic!

People in this category do not think in terms of the society in general, but rather they see themselves as standing alone in the world. They rely on their own inner source of authority, and they are desperate to satisfy their own wants or interests. The drug tourism literature on the internet and in advertisements speaks of the quest for creativity and personal growth, and of the need to be in tune with oneself. The inner domain and the importance of self-discovery and progress are frequently recurring themes. While there are thousands of different ways to explore inner reality, the hallucinogenic experience is quick. Illegal in the United States and Europe, it presents the lure of the dangerous or forbidden. Tourists are not interested in future salvation but self-actualization in the present.

Shamanic training is another theme that appeals to the tourists—they too can use their insights to help others. Heelas points out that many indeed emanate from the healing professions and find this kind of training very attractive, explaining why an individual might have three to four ayahuasca sessions in a week's time, when shamanic apprentices typically spread out such training over weeks or even months.

The plant is good for physiological arousal, heightened emotionality, and unusual sensations, especially because of the purging and diarrheas it provokes. Research by both de Rios and Masters and Houston[8] showed that 20 to 25 percent of individuals who took powerful LSD-like hallucinogens had a spiritual experience. This fits in with the quest of many of these people. Finally, the power of the hallucinogens to create a suggestible state is congruent with the shamanic environment—an all-powerful man (generally few women are involved, except perhaps in Brazil) who can direct the training, but who bows out after the week's dues are paid.

Criticisms of this phenomenon are easy to assemble. There are narcissistic, selfish, permissive men and women who put their own selves first and foremost. They are self-indulgent. There is the issue of out-and-out theft of the long-standing spiritual teachings and practices of others. Men and women select what they want and ignore anything that does not fit their model. In fact, a number of Europeans and Americans have become self-styled ayahuasca healers themselves, pushing aside their trainers. This is what Heelas says is a form of self-enlightenment achieved in a couple of hundred hours. Heelas appears to admire the quest he has documented. Most important to this discussion is the quality of the individuals who are attracted to the shamanic activity. They are often untrained, uneducated, and hungry to make money! They mix and match numerous plants without any concern for their toxic properties and cause distress and illness to many of their clients.

Data on the New Healers

Based on their interviews in 2006–2007, Rumrrill and de Rios found that 80 percent of the new ayahuasca healers are men, called *curanderos, ayahuasqueros,* or plant doctors. Their ages range between 40–60 years of age, with there being only a few older healers. There is no formal professional training, and healers focus mainly on psychosomatic or stress-related disorders. Few are influenced by Western scientific medicine. A majority learned from family members and friends who practice folk medicine. None of those interviewed were mystics or admitted to involvement in witchcraft or esoteric organizations like the Rosicrucians, popular throughout Latin America. All used ayahuasca as well as other plants, including toé and chiricsanango. None saw any danger from the use of ayahuasca by their clients and denied any problems with their clients' health. Many are entrepreneurs who travel around the world by invitation from sponsors in major world cities. Several maintain web pages, edit brochures, and manage tourism firms. Hotels throughout Amazonian cities and towns have a shamanic service where they contract with a local ayahuasquero to meet the requests of their guests. Clients come mostly from the United States and Europe.

Overall, ayahuasca is disappearing as a sustainable plant in the Amazon, and it is often replaced by tobacco use. Religious groups like the UDV carefully cultivate the ayahuasca plants they use to prepare their sacrament. Many of the new shamans lack the experience, appropriate personality, and requisite training for this traditional healing work. Many are unable to accurately diagnose the illnesses that their clients suffer, which is necessary for effective curing. Nor are they aware of important facts about drug interactions, for example, that ayahuasca, antibiotics and antidepressive drugs can cause client poisoning. As a result, sometimes a drug tourist's condition worsens, and the client has to be rescued and sometimes hospitalized.

Given the potency of the chemicals involved and the new shamans' lack of understanding about them, this drug tourism—hiding out under the guise of spiritual questing—calls out for regulation. Unlike traditional mestizo or indigenous use of the plants within a ritualized context—with knowledge being passed on through periods of long and rigorous apprenticeship—drug tourism in contemporary Peru and the Amazon region is merely a footnote to drug trafficking around the world.

Deconstructing (Drug) Tourism

Berg, in seminal work that deconstructs tourism,[9] describes the tourist who emanates from the first world, Western context. An individualist in search of authenticity and the exotic, the tourist is in quest of an experience in a foreign land, to elevate themselves spiritually and to be entertained. The individualist does not want anyone to tell him what to do and flees unpleasant aspects of modernity in the search for the "authentic and the real." What the tourist does not realize is that she has fallen into a tourist trap, where tourists are exploited by pseudo-events in the hands of new shamans, who provide ersatz experiences geared to stereotyped notions of what an authentic hallucinogenic experience abroad should be. The tourist is easily satisfied by pseudo-authenticity—and seeks this authenticity to gain insight into his/her own life. In fact, the tourist does not care much if the experience is real or fake. He just wants to have fun and escape from the patterns that he follows in his regular life. We then have a hyperreal experience, one more real than reality. The tourist's quest for authenticity is irrelevant. There is a real risk involved, as most of these new shamans are charlatans who do not screen their clients. Visitors may succumb to panic attacks, heart arrhythmias, increases in blood pressure, paranoid thoughts, or even death. While the tourist may be seeking personal transformation, he is playing with fire. What is not realized is that the spiritual experience is created to cater to such tastes. It is inauthentic, mimicking a watered-down, shamanic religious tradition that has no history of proselytization. The tourist returns home with a story of his hardships in the Amazon, which supposedly proves to his friends there that he has experienced spiritual growth. It is true that traditional cultures have used plant psychedelics for spiritual purposes—they have been used as well as for power and control, for political manipulation, to bond youth together as cohorts, and for divination.[10] While very much interested in ethical relativism, anthropologists are clear that they cannot impose the values of their own society on another. However, when faced with harmful and dangerous practices, it is important to provide some standard of judgment. A humanitarian standard that follows the Hippocratic Oath—physician, do no harm—seems to set a minimum requirement. Moreover, in the opinion of the authors, anthropologists have not taken into account the role that their studies of drug rituals have had on this ethical conundrum.

The Anthropologist and Drug Tourism: Mea Culpa

With this in mind, we will briefly examine one of the authors' record as a scholar of hallucinogenic rituals in cross-cultural perspective, to see how the diffusion of this esoteric material may have followed. In the summer of 1967, de Rios lived in the coastal rural community of Salas, Peru, funded by the Institute of Social Psychiatry at San Marcos University, Lima, to study traditional folk healing with a mescaline cactus, San Pedro (*Trichocereus pachanoi*). Subsequently, with a Peruvian psychiatrist she spent a year in Iquitos, Peru, funded by the Foundations Fund for Research in Psychiatry, to study the use of ayahuasca in folk healing. As a visiting scientist at the Smithsonian Institution in the summer of 1970, she helped to prepare an exhibition, "Towards Man's Understanding of Drugs." Over the years, she returned to Peru several times to work intensively with one folk healer, don Hilde. In the 1990s, she became part of a transnational research team, funded by the Heffter Foundation, to study the use of ayahuasca among adolescents, members of the Brazilian religion União do Vegetal, and for this work she visited Brazil on two occasions.

Over the last 39 years she presented more than 70 papers and talks on her research, in 15 different countries, as well as publishing widely in this area. It never occurred to de Rios that her work had diffused to a general drug-seeking public, until she began to be invited to a few conferences that were less academic, with committed, drug-seeking men and women eager to learn more about ayahuasca—in effect, the drug tourists described in this book. Over the years, occasional professionals, unsolicited, would tell her about their own drug experiences in South America, still very much on their minds and in their memories.

De Rios began to focus on the damaging aspects of this phenomenon in 1992, when a woman contacted and came to visit her, referred by a mutual acquaintance in Peru. By this time, de Rios had established clinical psychology credentials and was working part-time as a mental health counselor at the University of California–Irvine Medical Center, in addition to her duties teaching anthropology. The visitor explained that she had just returned from almost daily use of ayahuasca in Peru (not at all the way that traditional healers functioned), and that the she was continually "merging with the universe." It was clear that the uncontrolled use of the plants was precipitating this woman into a psychotic state. In the case of this visitor, the so-called healer she was working with knew very little about ayahuasca before he set himself up as a specialist. He has agents abroad seeking clients for him, he maintains a large retreat outside of Iquitos, and he travels widely in Europe and the United States.

Esoterism and the Revolt of the Masses

Since time immemorial, esoteric knowledge has always been known to carry certain risks. Huston Smith, the historian of religion, in 2005 wrote that all religious traditions have a wisdom-based esoteric dimension summarized by the phrase "Cast not your pearls before swine." He cites a Taoist saying, "Know ten things, tell nine," and argues that some things should not be flaunted to the public. There are truths which can only be distorted and misunderstood if they fall on uncomprehending ears. The Catholic Index is another example of the way that control over esoteric material has occurred historically, in the form of an index of prohibited books. It was said to combat the publication of pernicious writings causing great harm, destruction or death, or wicked meaning. This was done in conformity with the dogmas of the Catholic Church.

Are anthropologists in a position where they should set up their own Index? "What happens if I publish?" says the scholar. "Will foolish people put themselves in danger as they romanticize my scientific findings and apply them to their own lives?" This argument becomes more poignant when we look at Ortega y Gasset's comments in 1932. While the author considered himself a political liberal, he was highly distrustful of the masses, whom he believed should not and in fact, cannot, direct their own personal existence. To allow them to rule, in his opinion, was a grave error. He disdained the idea that the average man thinks that he is just like everybody else. As a pseudo-intellectual, he is unqualified, unqualifiable, and disqualified. Ortega argues that the mass man or woman acts directly outside of the law and believes he or she is exempt from restrictions. All that counts is the vital desire he or she has.

If we apply this approach to drug tourism, we can only conclude that the drugs and rituals are out there, ready to be used and exploited, in spite of interdiction of law. One's search for pleasure and well-being is of primary concern, and such "mass" or pseudo-intellectual people demand access to the drugs as if it were their natural right to do so. "One should abandon oneself calmly to one's self-spirituality." "No one is superior to anybody, and there are no limits in sight." This mass man imposes his own vulgar views without respect for or regard to others. His life loses all authenticity and it is transformed into a fiction. Lack of morality follows—to wit in this context, the mocking of drug laws. Anybody and everybody boasts of practicing it, and it's very hip to go abroad to have a drug trip without worry that governmental authorities will throw you in jail. This antinomian phenomenon brings back shades of the 1960s—going against the law with the connotation that individuals believe they can rise above the law, to be above and outside the law.

Drug tourism calls out for regulation, given the potency of the chemicals involved. A general global tendency with regard to drug regulation in recent years has been based on medical models. This includes rigorous controls and oversight of these powerful substances. It is hard to imagine actual regulation of ayahuasca and its additives in societies that are complicit in allowing such activities to occur, due to the economic benefits that accrue to some of their citizens. Certainly more information on the risks involved needs to be disseminated, so that the public indeed bewares.

An Opposite Point of View

Not everyone thinks drug tourism is a bad thing. Many writers are convinced that in this postmodern world, atheism and agnosticism are protected by strong lobbies including skeptics and scientists. They are quick to debunk religious ideology. In lieu of traditional religious membership, there is a New Age phenomenon which argues for a sincere search for spiritual connectedness among many in Western nations, including the United States, Europe, and Canada. Some writers argue that Westerners who look for traditional spiritual medicine like ayahuasca should not be called drug tourists. They are simply pursuing spiritual or therapeutic opportunities for themselves, an acceptable quest among large numbers of New Age men and women.

One anthropologist, Winkelman,[11] himself once present among a group of ayahuasca providers in Brazil, interviewed 15 men and women who had spent large sums of money to stay in a four-star hotel in Manaus. They were in search of ayahuasca experiences to meet their needs. Winkelman queried them about their motivations to participate in such sessions and about the benefits they believed they obtained. He looked for common motivations as well as benefits. His conclusions were that these men and women were seeking spiritual relations, personal spiritual development, and emotional healing; they desired as well to develop personal self-awareness. They wanted to connect with nature, which they saw as sacred, with God, spirits, plants, and natural energies; the ayahuasca experience provided this for them. Most of those interviewed spoke of their desire to obtain increased self-awareness, personal insights, and access to deeper levels of the self. This would enhance their personal development, as well as help them obtain a personal direction in life.

Another group of tourists to ayahuasca sessions in Iquitos were queried by a reputable ayahuasca healer, whom we interviewed. He was kind enough to share his clients' comments with us. Pseudonyms are used.

Five men and two women were present. They came from France, the United States, and Canada. One man, a dentist, had as his objective "to connect with nature and the Amazon rain forest, to find internal peace, and to know [his] private world." "When I take ayahuasca," he said, "I discover the world, I discover myself and understand my anguish and depression that I have been suffering since I was 15 years old." A French geographer told us that he seeks the cause of his problems and to discover the shamanic world. He takes ayahuasca to find his own sense of self, to experience the plant medicine, and to learn about indigenous knowledge. His motivation included curing his addiction to drugs, which had been accumulating for many years. He blamed the origin of his problems on his mother. Now he felt better and had a sense of his future. He enjoyed working with the ayahuasca healer and reaching his objectives, and he claimed to have a much better outlook on life.

Robert, a carpenter from the United States, wanted to come to the Amazon and meet the healer who he was sure would help him cure his illness. Some 20 years ago, he had an accident. He works with yoga to feel better. He wanted to understand the way the plants work and to find a cure for his illness and understand his problems. Now that he has taken the ayahuasca he feels much better, and he believes he has found what he was looking for. He will return home satisfied and hopes to come back again.

Stan, a French student, found the healer to help him understand clearly his mental and physical states and to experience the plant medicine. He wants to cure himself from the psychological problems that have bothered him for many years. He is a nervous man and very sensitive. This is the first time he has taken ayahuasca. Previously, he tried Western medicines for his depression, without any success. Since he was young, he was closed off into an interior world of his own. Now, he wants to know the curative power of the jungle plants and to learn from them. He feels better now, and he thinks the experience has been very positive. He is sure of himself and hopes some day to work with the plants again.

A young Frenchman working in construction came to the Amazon to cure his psychological problems and to find inner peace. His problems started five years ago, when he was working in Africa and experimenting with a powerful West African hallucinogen, Iboga. When he began his treatment with ayahuasca and other medicinal plants, the first week he did not feel any better and was feeling tricked because he was not improving. The following week, he quickly felt he was opening into a different world for himself, and his life took on another perspective toward the world. He felt liberated. He now feels very content and thanks the healer for the good work he did with him.

A young woman, Patricia, a French professor, was attracted by the mysticism of the rain forest and the idea of trying plant medicines. When she came to the healing center, it was to experience the plant. But, when she took it, she discovered many things inside herself and about the world in general

She realized she had stomach and intestinal problems and pains. From her work with the healer she found a place where she encountered internal peace. She has a better vision of the path she should now follow in her life.

The last visitor, Marie, was a Canadian student. She came especially to treat her throat cancer. She took ayahuasca to help herself and to experience the medicine. The healer treated her with ayahuasca and other plants. She returned to her country content with what she found, in this marvelous world of plants which has made her feel better.

*   *   *

As sincere as the supplicants might be in their personal quests, the charlatans in whose hands they placed themselves cause us to wonder about outcomes. There is simply no tradition of religious conversion in the history of shamanism which developed at the dawn of human history, unlike the Christian concept of spreading the gospel. The societies in question were small in scale, and were comprised of hunters and gatherers of the same ethnic backgrounds. There was minimal diversity among them in beliefs, values, and goals. Shamanism, the religion of these hunters and gatherers, depended upon the community's sense of wonder and awe regarding supernatural and preternatural access. Ecstatic trances and exceptional emotional states of consciousness were commonplace. These shamans insisted on having power and being in control, and they were believed by all to be able to call upon spirits of plants and animals to do their bidding, to ensure good health and successful hunts for their relatives. Diversity and interaction with strangers was minimal. In fact, it was rumored that the famous "ice man" found deceased in the European Alps probably had never ventured more than 15 miles or so from his home base during his lifetime.

The farce currently resulting from the borrowing of shamanic elements in a hodgepodge of cobbled mysticism verges on the ludicrous. Moreover, unlike shamanic specialists who devote their lives to the study of healing and metaphysical plants and techniques of influence, the current crew of neo-shamans are a suspicious lot and leave much to be desired. At best, they are simply inept and rely on luck so as not to harm their clients. At worst, they can provoke psychotic breakdowns and distress among their clients, as they fleece them out of substantial cash. Some of the women are seduced, raped, and discarded after their novelty to the healer wears off.

The occasional bad trip experienced by New Age drug tourists leads many to try to make sense of the experience and to learn from it. No doubt they do so because the bad trip experience occurs with some frequency. Perhaps guidelines for Westerners in this drug touristic enterprise need to be included in local guidebooks. Some think that a bad trip can heal the

Westerner, by bringing to conscious awareness the negative effects of what it is like to mature in America.[12] The seeker can become connected, embrace his bad trip, and learn from it. Others overidentify with their vision of the beliefs of traditional societies, and they urge individuals to establish contact with spirit allies and to integrate into their own knowledge base that knowledge they obtain from the bad trip. In this way, they can be critics of their own culture. They can stand up and be counted about alienation, narcissism, and greed, all part of our Western heritage. The bad trip can also negatively reinforce one's own past behaviors and the thoughts which drag us down. Long live the bad trip, so we can rise up from the ashes of our own destructive behavior, now removed, and be able to set forth on a new life journey.

Certainly, the bad trip has its share of commentaries in the New Age drug literature. From an anthropological point of view, assault sorcery and witchcraft in Amazonia is a theme that needs to be addressed here. There is indeed a dark side of shamanism. Belief exists in Amazonia about the use of psychic power derived from the plants being able to harm others through witchcraft machinations. This is a widespread theorem. De Rios documented this phenomenon in 1972,[13] when large numbers of men and women sought help from ayahuasca healers to remove witchcraft hexes. It was believed that the powerful ayahuasca healer could "work" to learn the cause of the witchcraft illness and then return the illness to its perpetrator. In the process, he would cure the client's illness.

The shaman in non-state-level societies was viewed as a moral arbiter of society. Mostly men, these shamans existed in a world of dualism, where good and evil were in a constant push-pull relationship. Common beliefs were that the shaman kills or harms his clients' enemies, to create retribution for their bewitchment. There is no simple path to the light, when forces out of harmony are everywhere in nature and are found among humans. This dual concept of good and evil in a delicate balance is current in many traditional societies, and it certainly is in Amazonia. The bad trip for Westerners can be attributed to a lack of a cultural tradition which sets up expectations, values, and beliefs for a given psychedelic experience. The setting of the experience as well as the dosage level of the hallucinogen play into this to enable us to predict the drug experience. Amazonian farmers who drink the ayahuasca tea report that they see the mother spirit of the vine, believed to be a boa constrictor, a fine hunter in its own right, moving quietly through the forest floor and trees to hunt its prey. A sign of healing is when the boa teaches the client its song. This is a harbinger of healing. For many Westerners, the only boa they have ever seen has been textile creations in scarves, in purses, or on a television nature special.

In many Amazonian traditional societies where psychedelics are taken, themes of death and resurrection are manifest. In tribal societies where shamans use plant drugs, individuals' relationships to their own society contrast dramatically with the individualism of Western society, which lacks any historic context for ingesting hallucinogens. Even in the old days, when Timothy Leary was out of control and was giving LSD to students and visitors, he was reputed to read from *The Tibetan Book of the Dead* to help structure the hallucinogenic experience for participants. In this way, he tried to avoid bad trips for participants. The Amazonian neo-shamans do not appear to have any theory about bad trips or their purpose. With the hodgepodge of nightshade plants that they mix in the brew, they simply are good at creating bad trips for their customers!

The Ayahuasca Seekers: Who Are They, and What are They Looking For?

The baby boomers' search for meaning and truth is witnessed by the explosion around the globe of new religions and diverse spiritual techniques. It should not surprise anyone that the Amazon is not exempt from attracting visitors who seek guidance and insight into personal problems, as well as help to alleviate the pain from what has been called "the empty self." Cushman, a psychologist,[14] has described the empty self of the post–World War II period, where individuals are soothed and filled up by consuming food, consumer products, and experiences. Since World War II and the advent of nuclear warfare and the potential for planetary destruction, individuals experience psychological states such as low self-esteem and confusion about their values. Drug excesses are a constant, and the Westerner is compelled to fill his emptiness with chemically induced emotional experiences.

Seguin wrote about the phenomenon of charlatan psychiatry.[15] This term was applied to a long tradition in Latin America of nonauthentic folk healers who had malicious and fraudulent intentions. They provided hallucinogenic plant drugs in ritual settings for their own personal gain. In Seguin's research, unscrupulous practitioners exploited their victims and were conscious of the farce in which they were involved. Today in California and elsewhere, there are zealots who devote their lives to a new age of drug use, and they urgently proselytize others to immerse themselves in drugs, "to make more, to use more, to sell more." Many are irresponsible and unconscionable individuals. In Peru and Brazil, in Amazonian cities and large towns, mestizo men become instant traditional healers without undergoing any apprenticeship period, without having any teachers and without control. The hallucinogenic plants in question have never been used traditionally in the way that the self-styled healers use them, and there are numerous psychological casualties.

Drug tourism is found on a somewhat smaller scale than international mass tourism and is shrouded in a special rhetoric. Travel literature includes terms like "advanced shamanic training," which is coupled with descriptions of healer so and so who has explored inner space, or other terminology to cue the tourist as to the actual meaning. Drug tourists perceive the natives as timeless and ahistoric. They do not recognize the vast worlds of change between the tribal native, the civilized Indian, the lower-class laborer, the striving middle-class individual, and the managerial elite of the Amazon region's major industries. Nor do the tourist guides have any interest in filling in all the shades of gray for them. Drug tourists are desperate to find the vanishing primitive. They cannot or will not see the urban and civilizing influences in these Amazon cities, including 400 years of Catholic and Protestant proselytization. They miss out on the movies, radio, television, schools, libraries, and other Western-type infrastructures everywhere. The Westerner is not involved in a native ritual of spiritual dimensions, as she has been led to expect, but is rather in a staged drama to turn her on and remove her cash.

In the tribal and industrialized societies for which data on hallucinogenic use are available historically, we see that access to supernatural power and the unitive or oceanic experience was highly valued. Hallucinogenic plants were used to enhance perception and intuition. These plants evoke spiritual experiences in at least 20 percent of a given population. Throughout de Rios' studies of traditional societies of the world that have utilized hallucinogens prior to the advent of drug tourism, she found that plant hallucinogens provided little, if any, abuse potential. Most of the plants were of limited availability and were given in religious ritual settings in natural environments with all the senses engaged. Elders and religious leaders were present in these ritual settings to ensure a smooth interior voyage, and those taking the hallucinogenics were laden with educational and didactic contact for reassurance. Hallucinogens have been used in a magical-religious context, with ceremony, to celebrate or contact the realm of the supernatural, and to divine the future, throughout human history. The power of mind-altering plants was acknowledged to belong to special realms constrained with taboos and rituals. Any one who entered those portals had to be properly prepared for the journey.

CHAPTER 4

THE NEW SHAMANS

If we look in general at the recent spate of neo-shamans, we see that most of these men and women are basically business people who extract cash from visitors. Today, drug tourist clients are not screened and new healers mix together toxic witchcraft plants of the nightshade family with ayahuasca. Most have never been apprentices, nor fasted, nor adhered to special diets that traditional healers typically have used to enhance their ability to understand the plant hallucinogenic effect. Moreover, the world is a different place than it was in the 1960s when de Rios conducted her research on ayahuasca use among mestizo men and women. Now, there are many foreign visitors with dietary and pharmacological restrictions interacting with the plant hallucinogens in a harmful way.

Charlatan healers are hardly new to the Peruvian scene. In a nation of almost 20 million inhabitants, there are less than 250 psychiatrists, and those who do exist practice in cities such as Lima, Arequipa, and so on. There are thousands of curanderos (folk healers), vegetalistas (herbalists), curiosos (fortune-tellers) or sanitarios (paramedics) who practice in cities and villages alike, who rub shoulders with well-touted witches (called brujos) as well as with occasional spiritualist healers.

The Peruvian psychiatrist Carlos Alberto Seguin studied the native therapy systems, and he clearly recognized that the natural history stage of data gathering was a first step before any cultural universals could be applied to understand the diversity of Peru's therapeutic panorama. He used the term "folk psychiatry" to comment on this popular realm. He defined it as the study of ideas, beliefs, and practices referring to the clinical picture of illness and its treatment that is maintained by popular tradition. This is in contrast to what is accepted by the dominant culture in which the system functions, in this case, Western biomedicine. Not only does this kind of folklore psychiatry treat mental illness, but it also looks at relevant factors such as socioeconomic, intellectual, legal, and religious traditions. This ethnopsychiatry studies cultural or ethnic groups in their own environment and defines concepts from the point of view of the native person. It is part of popular wisdom.

Another type of healing commonly found in Peru can be delineated, called charlatan psychiatry. This is certainly not limited to Peru, and indeed is found in underdeveloped countries throughout Latin America. Practitioners of folk psychiatry are authentic, while charlatans do not believe in what they say or do. They are commercially oriented, without scruples, and they mix popular ideas with pseudoscientific and pseudo-religious ones. They practice for pure economic gain and have been reported in diverse parts of the world. Academic psychiatrists in third world countries like Peru have become more and more distanced from their patients, and at the same time, there is a rise in the proliferation of charlatans, even when there is legal or police repression of such practices. The medicine man—in this book, the traditional mestizo healer—was an integral part of his community; the charlatan may not be. The mestizo healer plays a decisive role in the life of the group to which he belongs and has a definite role linked to the structure of the community. Generally respected, the medicine man is paid for his work. Women are generally delegated to the realm of witchcraft potions and matters of love, and not until menopause do we see female traditional urban healers exercising their practice.

The charlatan practices a scam, tricking his clients. He is not integrally linked to his public. He does not represent any clear-cut tradition. He may be intentionally malicious and fraudulent with personal economic gain being a sustaining motivation. In this chapter we see vignettes of all of these types, from indigenous Amazon basin healers to traditional shamanic healers to new-shamans.

We interviewed 15 of these new shamans over a two year period (26 shamans, if we include those of indigenous ethnicity). Many of the supposed shamans are people without experience, with sociopathic tendencies, who do not have the personal capacity, preparation, or personality for this work. They simply traffic in plant hallucinogens. Many do not know how to cure. They cannot diagnose the illnesses that many clients bring to the healing session. On occasion, madness or death has followed when the new shamans add toxic plants, often in the nightshade family, to the mixture. Drug interactions also cause problems as antibiotics, antidepressive medications, and even dairy products interact with the ayahuasca or other additives and poison the client.[1] The Centers for Disease Control inform us that in the United States, 10 percent of adult women and 4 percent of adult men take antidepressant medications.[2] This would certainly impact tourists from North America at any ayahuasca session.

Some seekers complain about the jungle hotels of numerous centers of ayahuasca healing along the highway to Nauta in Iquitos. Many foreign visitors are picked up right off the plane in Iquitos, rushed to the healing center, and immediately given ayahuasca before they even acclimate to the heat and change of climates from coastal Peru to the rain forest. Some healers give daily subeffective doses of the hallucinogens to gradually build up to the amount of a full dose. Some of the ceremonies have as many as 30 people taking ayahuasca at once. This occurs when large groups come for two-week-long, intensive so-called "seminars" to learn about the plants, to enter into a diet, and to take ayahuasca. Even the most popular and respected healers do not always take precautions to avoid overdoses or contraindications of the ayahuasca. The visitors blindly trust the healer to know what is best for them. Such an approach does not always work and may be dangerous. There is no basic harm reduction information about what the client should expect from the ayahuasca, what kind of physical effects they will feel during the process. One scholar in Iquitos has told us that ayahuasca should not be taken until eight months after the last dose of a antidepressive medication. Even the National Institute of Health in Iquitos is considering starting a work group to distribute harm reduction pamphlets to travel agencies and other tourist gathering places in Iquitos, Pucallpa, and Tarapoto to alert tourists to common dangers.

Data on the New Shamans

Younger healers are as prestigious as older ones and, as entrepreneurs, they often live in cities. Some have college educations and travel widely outside of Peru. They give conferences, publish books, and replace the older healers—certainly they do not work as apprentices to them. Those shamans who come from rural backgrounds were farmers and extracted forest products by hunting and fishing before they decided to become healers. Those from urban backgrounds had a history of precarious occupations. Many were day laborers or street peddlers. None of the new healers have had formal professional training, and they focus mainly on treatment of psychosomatic or stress-related illnesses. Few of them have been influenced by or know much about Western scientific medicine. The majority of them learned their trade from family members or friends who practiced healing. All have incorporated ayahuasca into their practice, as well as other plants like toé and chiricsanango. They are generally unfamiliar with the more than 4,400 plants known and used by indigenous peoples and rural farmers. Those in cities with mestizo heritage have a much lower fund of knowledge about plants than indigenous healers. Of the new mestizo shamans, many hold beliefs permeated by esoteric and spiritualist currents. Many introduce modern elements like dancing and music to the healing ceremonies.

The healers deny that any danger occurs from the use of ayahuasca, although rumors abound in the cities and countryside about deaths that suddenly occurred among ayahuasca users from heart attacks, aneurysms, and other similar problems. It is possible that the ayahuasca plant will become extinct with time, as it appears to be disappearing as a sustainable plant in the Amazon. Tobacco is replacing ayahuasca use in many indigenous areas of Peru.

These new shamans are entrepreneurs who travel around the world by invitation. They have clients in New York, Vienna, Vancouver, Amsterdam, and elsewhere. They maintain web pages and edit brochures touting their talent and expertise. Brochures are full of verbiage proclaiming all-inclusive shamanic workshops that provide "sacred ayahuasca drinks." They offer hiking trails, swimming, piranha fishing, boat excursions, bird watching, and access to exotic and colorful wildlife. They "guarantee" that the shamans are native (it is unclear what they mean by this) and often throw in other New Age activities like chakra therapy, shamanic guided journeys, drumming, breathing exercises, and the like. The plants are said to bridge the mundane and spiritual worlds and cause a transformation for the individual to a time and a place where traditional beliefs remain intact.

Our research shows a lack of communication and respect between doctors and curanderos. Both sides exhibit a negative attitude toward the other. Doctors never advise a patient to seek the help of a curandero; de Rios observed this to be the case in 1968–1969. It is paradoxical that patients tended to visit a curandero only after years of failed treatment if they were suffering from a psychosomatic disease; similarly, some patients end up in a hospital with confusion and disorientation after numerous unsuccessful ayahuasca ceremonies.

On the other hand, some curanderos send their patients to hospitals for checkups or treatment. This is beneficial for both the healer and the patient and should be encouraged. However, the opposite is almost never true. Doctors, with very few exceptions, do not advise their patients to seek the help of a curandero.

In Iquitos there are a number of nonprofit groups conducting scientific research on the healing properties of plants, but not enough, and there is virtually no financing. There are a large number of visitors that some local people call "narco-tourists," especially in Iquitos. Virtually every foreigner who is there is on a three-day- to a three-week-long "ayahuasca trip," without even knowing the significance of the ceremony or the biological functions of the ayahuasca drink. There are at least 10 establishments offering "viajes espirituales" (spiritual voyages) in Iquitos. The same phenomenon to a lesser degree occurs in Pucallpa and Tarapoto, Peru.

A prevalence of charlatans emphasize the recreational properties of ayahuasca and charge much larger sums than usual. They attempt to advertise themselves by belittling other shamans. About two out of three mestizo curanderos turn out to provide pure tourist entertainment. Many foreigners in Peru, for example, have a personal story to tell connected to curanderos. Virtually everyone believes in curanderismo enough to have visited one at least once, with varying results. The town of Iquitos is full of troublesome rumors of tourists who have overdosed on ayahuasca. The outcome is psychological instability and, in one recent case, even the death of a Swedish student. Ayahuasca is also exported abroad and said to be mixed with opium, in illegal drug trade. The boundaries between the shamans and the charlatans are not drawn finely enough. Many agree that the charlatans need to be controlled and their practices prohibited. In addition, racism in all spheres of life is rampant, including relationships between indigenous and mestizo curanderos. In the following accounts, pseudonyms will be used.

Don Alberto from Pucallpa

Alberto is 37 years old and has been practicing curanderismo since he was 14. He treats mostly the local population who suffer from physical ailments, but sometimes they may also have psychological disorders. Alberto prescribes various plants for his clients and sometimes, but not always, supplements this with ayahuasca ceremonies. He claims that he is able to cure every known disease with a specific plant. The plants come to him in ayahuasca visions after he comes across a patient with a new disease. Very often, the medicinal plants can be found in every kitchen: Alberto cures leukemia using plantains, and he treats prostate issues with the skin of the pineapple. There are very few overlaps between these remedies compared to the plants used by Arrévalo. If Alberto sees that he will not be able to cure a patient, he sends him/her away. In this way he claims he never had a patient who died after his treatment. Alberto urges the patient to visit a hospital every two weeks to take tests that monitor the course of his or her disease. He ends the healing only after the patient is healthy again.

This healer spent four years as a military psychologist. He admits that the training as a psychologist allows him to generate confidence and, in this way, to begin his patient's cure. In his own words, "conversation takes away half of the disease." He started learning when he was 14 (he is now in his thirties) and answered "a call" to look for plants and try them out on himself. He then went through the usual two-year apprenticeship and continued his studies in an "Occult Science School" in Brazil under the guidance of a teacher. He admits that he also learned a lot during the four years he spent as an army detective, when he received training as a psychologist. This now allows him to better listen to his patients' needs. According to Alberto, it takes only one ayahuasca ceremony to discover a cure for a new disease—the ayahuasca shows him which plant will heal.

Benjamin

This healer started when he was 24 years old (he is now in his mid-thirties), after the death of his father. He always mentions his deceased father with special respect and love. Before that, he used to be a teacher. He went through a two-year apprenticeship. He now has a school for *sabios viejos* (wise elders), where the local curanderos can exchange knowledge and experience, and they can talk about and learn to be responsible with patients. Benjamin is helped with the school by his brother Rogelio, who is also a curandero.

David

One healer is involved as president of a local group called AIDESEP (Asociación indígena por el desarrollo de la Selva Peruana, or Indigenous Association for the Development of the Peruvian Rain Forest). David is in his early forties and worked as a teacher for 12 years. He then decided to go through apprenticeships to become "a spiritual guide," as he calls it. Now he has finished three years out of seven years' training in total. David has been thinking about establishing a medical school, where the traditional and Western medicines would be combined. He has actually started a pilot class that is going to graduate this year.

Eduardo

Another healer, Eduardo, started to heal when he was about 20 years old. He went through the "normal" apprenticeship with a local healer in Iquitos. Eduardo reports that he started learning at about 16 years of age and began curing at 20; he was taught by his uncle, father, and grandfather. Curander-ismo is a family tradition, so now Eduardo is teaching his skills to his 14-year-old son. He emphasizes the practical part of the apprenticeship: being a "nurse" for the maestro. He believes that people keep on learning their whole life, especially because it is necessary to find a cure for every new disease. The more complicated the disease, the longer it takes to figure out the right plants to use for patients. For instance, he has already spent 10 years looking for the cure for AIDS and still has not found it. By comparison, Alberto claims that one ceremony is enough to find a plant to use against any new disease, even one as complicated as leukemia, which he cures with bananas.

Federica

A female healer, Federica—one of the few—began healing when she was 16 years old. Among traditional healers, women were excluded from ayahuasca sessions when they were menstruating. Doña Federica told us that she was sick with some fatal illness (she would not disclose exactly which illness), and she said she was cured by a local shaman. Then she became interested herself in healing and went through a year of apprenticeship with the same shaman. All the time she went against her mother's wishes, as she wanted to see Federica become a lawyer.

Don Jorge from Pucallpa

This healer is 35 years old and has been working for 11 years at the outskirts of Pucallpa, treating local people and tourists in about equal proportion. He works with two brothers and a cousin. The ceremony is led by four shamans who sing icaros together, which, according to Jorge, allows them to join their powers together. It also creates an incredible experience for the participant. Don Jorge cures with ayahuasca ceremonies and ointments made from other medicinal plants; he also uses some massages. He always emphasizes the responsibility of a curandero, who must get to know the patient, the disease, and the previous treatment before he begins the healing process for them. Jorge must modify the ayahuasca dose based on each individual and on each disease and should be cautious about which tourists he admits into the session. Don Jorge has a degree in education, which has influenced his healing. He has established a "school of wisdom" where he teaches healing, responsibility, and ethics to new apprentices and experienced curanderos. Also, this is a way to share experiences between curanderos. He has compiled a dictionary of Shipibo terms used in icaros, most of which have already been forgotten even by the curanderos who sing them.

Don Nestor from Yurimaguas

This healer is about 60 years old and has been working since his childhood. He treats the local people and takes tourists on a two-day- to three-month-long "retreat" in the jungle. He uses various plants in both tobacco and ayahuasca ceremonies. He diagnoses by taking the patient's pulse and by employing the power of suggestion. In one diagnostic ceremony, he gradually convinced the patient that she had a headache with dizziness, and a sore throat. At the beginning of the evening, the patient was complaining of nothing of the sort. Nestor has a good reputation in this small jungle city. Several patients claim to have been healed by him. He is not too careful about the doses of ayahuasca that he gives, and he allows the patients take as many glasses as they wish, although two are usually enough. Don Nestor has emphasized the recreational aspect of ayahuasca visions, stressing the beautiful aerial voyages, the bright colors, and so on.

Other Healers Along the Way

There is don Pedro from Tarapoto. He was a high-level administrator of a coastal university and has been a curandero for at least 25 years. He maintains his own center close to Tarapoto and admits mostly tourists from the United States. Don Pedro travels frequently to southern California and has written a book of poetry. At a ceremony to announce the book's publication, he appeared dressed in Jívaro shaman gear from Ecuador. He sang icaros to the people gathered in the Tarapoto municipality building, and he held a plastic bottle containing ayahuasca while he read his poetry.

A second self-proclaimed healer, don Ricardo, is from Yurimaguas, Peru. Supposedly, he works with plants and is an ayahuasquero. He keeps a mix of Inca, Buddhist, and Christian paraphernalia in his study and claims to be "the best in the world." He states that "all these Indians are liars." He charges about three times more than any other curandero. When talking about plants, he is unable to list any medicinal properties. He has very few visitors and is considered to be a charlatan among the local mestizo people.

A third man, don Esteban from Yurimaguas, is a Brazilian who cures with the help of the Virgin Mary and the saints. He uses plants and tobacco. To diagnose, he takes two colorful ropes and a mirror and spends at least five minutes trying to convince those present that they have stomach aches, which may or may not be true. He has very few patients.

Don Salvador, Iquitos

This healer is mestizo with indigenous roots. His father was from the Cocama tribe in the south central Amazon region. At 60 years of age, he has had some 30 years of experience. Don Salvador maintains a center close to a tribal community where he has spent all his life. He cures with ayahuasca ceremonies and utilizes various plants. The price for foreigners is $50 per night, while the price for locals depends on the illness and what he feels like charging. At any one time he may have between one and ten people in the center. Local people usually come to be cured of physical ailments, while foreigners suffer from depression, anxiety, or drug addiction. Don Salvador cures cultural illnesses like daño and hexes due to witchcraft of evil people. These illnesses, according to him, are very difficult to treat and are incurable if the disease is well advanced. He used to work in the Takiwasi Center in Tarapoto, Peru a few years ago but now cures alcoholism and drug addiction on his own. Recovering addicts usually spend six months to one year in his center and are given very strong detoxifying plants. They also participate in ayahuasca ceremonies. Don Salvador encourages them to work in his farm to learn to appreciate their own work and thus to build up their self-confidence. His treatment also includes physical rehabilitation. He currently has a patient who was sent out of a hospital with half of her body paralyzed as the result of a stroke. After two months of saunas and massages at his center, the only part of the patient's body that remained paralyzed was her left foot, and the healer expected complete recovery within the next month or so. He believes that it is always useful to consult medical doctors or refer patients to them, especially when the disease is acute. However, he stresses the importance of examining the patient thoroughly before making a diagnosis, whether it is a medical doctor or a healer.

Don Salvador is not religious, although he was brought up Catholic. In addition to healing, he also has taken up sustainable agriculture and maintains a rather large farm for the region, about 20 acres. He grows yucca, sacha-papa (a starchy plant), and bananas for his personal use. There are also a few medicinal plants he tends, and there are about six acres of cacao for market sales. Don Salvador proudly points to his farm's good yields during successive years with relatively little harm to the environment. He is constantly looking for projects and financial aid to use his own farm as an educational tool for other members of the community or for elementary-school children to visit and learn from.

Doña Berta, Iquitos

This woman healer comes from an unusual ethnic background. Her father was born in the Brazilian Amazon, and her mother in the Andes. Quechua (the language of the ancient Inca) was the language she spoke at home. Both of her parents hail from families of healers, so she learned to combine traditional Amazonic and Andean healing methods in her practice. She is 42 years old and has been working for almost 23 years. Two years ago she established her own center on the major highway from Iquitos to Nauta. She charges about $15 for a diagnosis and $200 for a week's stay in the center. She also heals local people in Iquitos in her house in the city, charging much lower rates. She is adept at the use of plants and diagnoses with tobacco. About 10 years ago she began to perform ayahuasca ceremonies. She worked with another ayahuasquero at his center where, according to doña Berta, she had to do most of the hard work. She tried to treat some patients that her teacher would send away. She saved up enough money to establish her own place.

The center is frequented by local people as well as foreigners who suffer from various illnesses. Two ayahuasca tourists showed up, but doña Berta promptly asked them to leave. Overall, she is very conscious of the number of tourists in and around Iquitos and is very skeptical of most healers she knows in Iquitos. She emphasizes that the plant itself (and not "a plant spirit") cures a disease; her knowledge of plants and their functions is matched perhaps only by that of don Guillermo Arrévalo, among the curanderos that we have interviewed. Doña Berta does not believe in the witchcraft hexes either, but rather she believes that every disease has a physical cause. Overall, doña Berta has a very practical view of folk healing as her profession rather than as a sacred activity.

She uses various plant drinks, patches to cure skin infections and fungi, baths and massages to treat her clients' depression. During the ayahuasca ceremony she always starts out giving her clients a small dose and gradually increases it. She is conscious of the potential contraindications with ayahuasca.

Doña Rosalia, Huasco, Peru (near Cuzco)

This female healer uses coca and presents an interesting comparison to the other healers mentioned in this chapter. Like most ayahuasqueros, she works with local plants, but she uses coca leaves to diagnose diseases. She holds ceremonies where she offers thanks to Pachamama ("mother earth") and asks for her protection. Unlike with ayahuasca healers, no one, neither the healer nor the visitor, consumes coca during the ceremonies. She is 55 years old and has been working for 11 years. She is an Andean native and a Quechua speaker. She says she learned to heal from her husband and mother-in-law during her years of apprenticeship. Now she hopes that one of her granddaughters will become a curandera as well. Aside from a few women ayahuasqueros, healers we interviewed are generally male. By contrast, coca curanderos seem to be mostly female, a least the most respected ones. There is always a line of local people waiting in front of her door to be seen. She also accepts tourists as clients. She mostly cures various stomach ailments, psychosomatic diseases, headaches, depression, and anxiety.

She admits that she cannot cure cancer, heart diseases, or chronic illnesses, and she sends patients to the hospital instead when they present with these illnesses. However, she also believes that the hospital treatment, although faster, does not cure the disease entirely; while traditional treatments last much longer and are less pleasant, nonetheless, they eradicate the disease completely.

Dona Rosalia uses the same mixture of plants for any disease she is asked to heal, because she says there will always be one plant that is going to work. She admits she does not know exactly which plant will cure which disease. Additionally, she reads the coca leaves, which is very similar to diagnosing with tobacco, a practice used by many ayahuasqueros. Doña Rosalia concentrates on shuffling coca leaves, much like tea leaf readings, to give very generalized statements about her clients' lives.

Prices Charged by Healers

These charges vary enormously, from $40–$50 at Guillermo Arrévalo's center, to $1,000–$1,500 per month at Takiwasi for a nine-month period. Alberto charges according to the disease, which price usually does not exceed 100 soles. One healer charges 50 soles a ceremony, but visitors are invited to imbibe for free the first time. Eduardo charges $35, and visitors are invited for free the first time. At Federica's, the cost is $40–$45 for both patients and visitors. It appears that when a fixed rate is collected by an individual healer, it is more likely to be a case of a charlatan at work. The traditional technique, like that of don Hilde, is "pay me after you see the good results," which is how several healers treat their local patients, but not tourists. Curanderos who have centers in the rain forest charge more than those who work in the city. Similarly, tourists always pay more for their experience than local men and women. That does not mean that all curanderos who accept tourists are charlatans, since maintaining a healing center is expensive.

Doña Eugenia, Iquitos

This healer on the highway to Nauta, outside of Iquitos, keeps a very strict discipline in her center, and she does not allow alcohol there or permit romances to develop. She uses aromatherapy to cure depression, anxiety, and individuals' low self-esteem; she includes baths with flower petals and extracts, as well as massages using strong-smelling fruit lotions. According to her, aromatherapy tends to work best for women. Eugenia is a Catholic and works as an oration healer. She says she cures only with her songs, or icaros, that address plants as well as God and the Virgin Mary. She does not invoke animal spirits such as those of the Cocama curanderos. She describes the glory of Catholic-type heaven in her chants addressed to God. The songs are very melodic, energetic, and celebratory-sounding, not like those of other curanderos. Eugenia likes to express her joy at curing and to give thanks to God for the ayahuasca.

Sexual Activities and Abuse Issues in the Ayahuasca Centers

Among the curanderos, rumors abound regarding the sexual abuse of female clients while they are under the effects of ayahuasca (as one healer points a finger at another). There is a particular healer famous for his "moves" on female clients, including out-and-out rape. Women tourists feel safe taking ayahuasca with Federica, the female healer, in her place of business, perhaps explaining her popularity. However, one of the tourists interviewed complained about being touched in a sexual manner by one of Federica's male assistants. Some healers forbid romances between visitors, or even alcohol. At some centers, however, visitors bring their own drinks and combine partying and ayahuasca ceremonies. Dating is not uncommon between visitors in almost all the other centers we interviewed. Finally, the disdain with which some healers view their clients is personified in a story of a healer who used his cell phone during the ceremony and left at midnight although the patients were still high on the ayahuasca. They had to finish up their visions and find their way home in the wee hours of the night.

Dosage Levels

These also vary quite a bit. At Arrévalo's center, everyone receives almost the same, except children and patients who may have had a very strong reaction to ayahuasca. These latter individuals start with a spoonful before bed every night, whether there is a ceremony or not, and then can increase the dosage. However, for this protocol to be followed, they need to have had a negative experience first! The second and even the third doses are easier afterwards. The healer makes sure to avoid contraindications with medicine (checking out prior use of antidepressive medications, any heart problems, and so on). Another healer did not mention or inquire about health issues of patients and was uninterested in any potential contraindications. One healer treats his patients for two days without them taking ayahuasca. He then gives the patient a small dose and gradually increases it. He is very serious about the responsibility of the shaman and tries to avoid contraindications. In case of a bad trip, it takes about three weeks of "cleaning" work before the patient can take ayahuasca again. One healer in Yurimaguas uses the same dosage for all and pays no attention to contraindications. He is quick to double the dose if the visitor wishes to have stronger visions. Another healer in Iquitos gives small doses and repeats it once if there is no effect. He tries to avoid contraindications.

Another Iquitos healer starts with a small, subclinical dose and gradually increases it. If it is going to be a one-time experience, then he advises the client to try a full dose. He makes sure to explain the preparation and effects of ayahuasca to his visitors beforehand. Federica gives the visitor as much as he wants, so the second dose comes along very easily. The healer does not ask her patients about contraindications and leaves it for them to beware of such. Recently she had a case when she visited Holland where a woman patient on antidepressants experienced a very bad trip.

Profile of Foreign Visitors to Ayahuasca Sessions

Data were gathered on some of don Guillermo's patients in September 2007. There were eight people present from France, two from the United States, and one each from Belgium, Australia, Italy, Israel, Spain, Germany, and Canada. Ten were women and seven men. Their ages were between 23 and 37. Many expressed personal problems, including a lack of direction in life—the most commonly expressed by far. Also, many suffered from depression, anxiety, low self-esteem, eating disorders, post-traumatic disorders, and drug abuse.

Everyone had tried at least one psychedelic drug before the ayahuasca session, usually psilocybin or LSD. One individual had also tried peyote, and another the mescaline cactus San Pedro. Three had actually taken ayahuasca in their home settings. Needless to say, everyone had a history of smoking marijuana. Several had tried ecstasy and cocaine. One visitor was there after a long-term abuse of various drugs.

Many were looking for love, compassion, or they wanted to work individually with the shaman. They mainly sought tranquility. Their complaints were that not enough time was spent with the curandero and that there were lots of self-centered people together in the center, with not enough love or compassion within the group. They also complained about the touristic atmosphere.

Other Voices: Professionals Speak Out

Interviews were held with professionals in Iquitos and Tarapoto, Peru to obtain their reaction to this drug tourism phenomenon. One physician showed great interest in ayahuasca and has himself interviewed a number of healers about how they determine dosage, and about problems that arise when the tea is given to people without much knowledge of their prior health conditions. The physician measured participants' pulses, breath rate, and blood pressures during an ayahuasca ceremony. Although he never published his findings, he stated that after one to two hours of the ayahuasca ceremony, the blood pressure, pulse, and breath rate increased and only returned to normal some four hours later. There were also some dangerous contraindications for patients who were on antidepressive medications, because of a flooding of a brain chemical, serotonin,[3] which causes an overload and possibly severe depression subsequently. The physician suggested that individuals avoid these medications for as long as eight weeks before they participate in any ceremony.

He was also very adamant about avoiding what he called fake healers. He had his own list of good guys out in the community, but these names did not always match the opinions of other professionals. His greatest complaint about the charlatans in Iquitos is that they do not pay enough attention to the patient's health condition or to any medicine that the patient has taken prior to participation in the ceremony. This physician said that other professionals in the city have little beliefs in the efficacy of traditional medicine. This doctor planned to work with biochemists from Europe in the next few years, to examine the effects of ayahuasca depending on gender, weight, age, and diagnosis of illness.

A second physician has more training in phytochemistry and is interested in the chemical properties of Amazonian plants. His work, however, has not as yet been published, although he has been working in this area for more than 20 years. He has studied the chemical properties of the healers' plants and stated that even the native peoples do not believe that their herbal remedies work anymore. They prefer Western medicine rather than preparations from plants to treat common ailments. For example, he gave one man a plant called *ojé* to get rid of worms (helminthic disease), and the man asked instead for a pill. This physician believes in the curative properties of plants. He mentioned many cases of false and harmful beliefs that abound in traditional medicine. His hope is that communication will increase between physicians and healers to combine the best of both practices. His understanding of ayahuasca treatment is that it is like psychotherapy, which helps a patient resolve past traumatic experiences and end up with feelings of love and tranquility. He truly believes that most healers sincerely hope that their patient will get better, an attitude he does not think occurs among Western-style physicians. The curandero's patient, in his opinion, has to work consciously to be healed, as opposed to being a passive recipient of medicine. The physician opposes the combination of indigenous ceremonies with Catholicism or mixing any kind of religion with science and medicine.

A woman professional biologist from Iquitos is interested in medicinal plant research at the Instituto de Investigaciones de la Amazonia Peruana (Peruvian Institute of Amazonian Research). She is author of various books about the plants and traditional medicine in the Amazon; she has been collecting the information from various curanderos over the years. She thinks that 90 percent of them are charlatans, who do not know much and also do not care to learn more—only to extract cash from the tourists. She has heard firsthand accounts about some curanderos who have been sexually harassing female visitors. In the past, she has tried to lead seminars and conferences for the curanderos to learn from each other, but very few show up. Similarly, she has tried to unite them in an association of vegetalistas (plant doctors), but the organization has never been officially established. Even the president and vice president of it do not get involved in the association—there is a lack of interest in such an organization. One of the issues has to do with the fact that some curanderos claim they are "the best" or better than others. She has invited everyone to these events, including the charlatans. Whatever serious medical research on ayahuasca exists has not been available to researchers in the region. She cited the fact that we do not even know what species of *Banisteriopsis* (of which there are 23 endemic in Peru) correspond to which kind of ayahuasca, since they have vernacular names such as "cielo," "lucero," "trueno," "negro," "amarrillo," and so on. Besides, she stated that she had seen a single article published in pharmacology journals or at similar levels, and there is a lack of long-term studies of the effects of ayahuasca in treating drug addiction or other mental health conditions.

One professional interviewed receives patients who believe that their illnesses are caused by *brujería* (witchcraft). They usually suffer from anxiety, panic, aggression, and depression. Many patients go to this healer after they have gotten worse when their relatives took them to a number of different curanderos. Some have severe mental illnesses like schizophrenia. They believe in the power of a brujo to cause disease, given the difficult social conditions under which they live. These patients are usually the poorest and most marginalized in the city. Therefore, their instability, suggestibility, and feelings of stress and aggression toward more favored members of society impair their immune response. Their bodies lose the natural defense mechanisms when they face what they believe to be the power of a witch. This physician believed in parapsychology but was hesitant to go into details. Some of his patients firmly dislike curanderos, because the ayahuasca ceremonies have made their conditions worse. This physician is preferred by his clients since his medicine has helped them lead a normal life.

Dr. Jacques Mabit, Tarapoto, Peru

This French physician, Jacques Mabit, is director of the Takiwasi Center for Drug Addict Rehabilitation and Research on Traditional Medicines in the Amazon city of Tarapoto, Peru.[4] The center treats alcoholism and drug addiction with an unusual twist. Dr. Mabit has been in the field for 15 years and was trained and licensed as a physician in France. He started Takiwasi because, according to him, he was told to do so in an ayahuasca vision he had. There are usually about 15 patients at a time in his center, and clients stay for at least nine months. Five times a year he holds seminars for people interested in traditional medicine. The program includes three weeks of intense dieting, ceremonies, and conferences. There are about 40 staff members, who include psychotherapists, doctors, and researchers obtaining their PhD or working on some kind of research project.

Mabit sells well-known healing plants such as *sangre de grado, uña de gato,* and others. He has a laboratory on the premises, but so far the only experiments are to control the quality of the products. His plans for the future include experiments to determine appropriate dosage levels of ayahuasca and the reaction of patients to different plants. Takiwasi mixes Catholic ritual with traditional medicine. In the large structure used for gatherings (maloca), there are icons of the Virgin Mary. Mabit sings icaros directed to Christian saints. There are two chapels and an altar, and Mass is given before an ayahuasca ceremony. According to Mabit, it is symbolism that is already familiar to the patients in a country with strong Roman Catholic influences, and this facilitates the healing process for them.

Each patient's dosage and treatment is personally adjusted. Mabit combines psychotherapy, yoga, massage, work tasks connected to living in a community, dieting, and ingesting various plants. He emphasizes the importance of the patient's motivation, and he claims that he has a 60 percent success rate. He is the first to admit, however, that until recently, he has not done long-term follow-up studies.

Ayahuasca has been known to the indigenous peoples of the Amazon for at least 8000 years. The concept of using one drug plant to treat another as a form of redemption is part of a harm reduction approach. Mabit's work actively incorporates ayahuasca in the treatment of drug addicts. Controlling the preparation, prescription, and psychotherapeutic follow-up brings about therapeutic benefits without causing the clients' dependence on the plant.

Compared to Western medicine, indigenous medicines have been seen to be effective, low cost, and culturally resonant with traditional beliefs of the mestizo populations treated. Mabit has been very impressed with the curanderos that he has met and observed, whom he saw as being effective in their treatment of physical, psychological, and psychosomatic illnesses that did not respond to conventional medical approaches. In particular, the shamanic use of altered states with or without plant medicines was an essential aspect of healing rituals. Holism is the keyword here, as the healers worked simultaneously on the physical, psychological, and spiritual levels of their patients. In Peru, there is a National Institute of Traditional Medicines which investigates traditional healing techniques and recognizes the vast potential of the resources available among the country's indigenous shamanic healers. When de Rios and Rumrrill visited one ayahuasca healer in Iquitos in 2007, they were able to tour his botanical garden, which was laden with healing plants for all types of physical and psychological illnesses.

For many years, Peru was a foremost producer of the coca plant, which can cause addiction to the free base of cocaine. Since the 1960s, however, Peru has become a major drug-consuming country. The toxic residues from the solvents used to extract pure cocaine from the leaf produce a type of paste that when smoked is highly poisonous because of the solvent residues, which are addictive and destructive to the individual and are often likened to crack cocaine. The number of professional rehabilitation treatment centers in Peru are minimal, and most are in the capital city of Lima. By default then, outside of large urban centers it falls upon the indigenous and traditional healers to treat these problems. Such healers were particularly successful in treating alcohol addiction, and as many as 60 percent of healers' patients resolved their addiction using the San Pedro cactus in the Peruvian coast, which contains a high amount of mescaline.

Most of the healers claim their powers come to them through dreams and the teachings of the plants themselves. The healers told Mabit that foreigners could learn as well, but they had to follow traditional rules, including special diets, isolation in the forest, and sexual abstinence. The spirits of the plants, along with the boa, would come and speak to the person. Mabit found himself in a quandary, since his training in medicine taught him that science means observable facts, a rigorous methodology, experimentation, and measurement. Healers, on the other hand, put aside the pretense of strict objectivity to adopt a knowledge system where subjectivity is all important. Mabit turned to self-experimentation for his training with ayahuasca. He began working regularly with ayahuasca and drug addicts. In addition to the ayahuasca plant, tobacco played an important role. Recent research on tobacco smoke shows that it can be used to evoke dopamine responses through secondary smoke, affecting the dopamine neurochemical that controls pleasure. The curanderos that Mabit worked with used purgative and psychoactive plants, which he called "teacher plants," in the isolation periods in the jungle that were part and parcel of the healers' trainings. The diets were considered to be essential for the apprentice. Needless to say, Mabit ran into difficulties with the medical establishment, where the traditional wisdom concerning recovery from alcohol or drug addiction is either complete abstinence or at the least, harm reduction. Such an approach focuses primarily on damage control and not on the healing of the individual's problems. The approach followed by Mabit looks at the spiritual needs and the quest for meaning of the individual, even when these are not formulated by the patient. While the person is encouraged to be responsible for his life and to be able to quit drugs, getting at a sense of meaning in life is important.

Mabit tried to tackle drug addiction from a radical new perspective. The well-known psychologist Ronald Siegel[5] has written about the drive of human beings to seek out alternative states of consciousness. These are seen as a fourth major instinctual drive among all animal species. Siegel has documented hundreds of cases where animals seek out and consume natural psychoactive substances. De Rios, too, in her cross-cultural studies has explored beliefs that animals teach human beings about hallucinogenic plants. The history of religions shows a large number of techniques used to altered normal waking consciousness, including dreams, trauma, orgasm, extreme physical exercise, extreme pain, fasting, prayer, meditation, yoga, and so on. In particular, individuals using these techniques often develop a sense of the ineffable—a strong sense of meaning to life that often follows these experiences. Mabit calls this "an attempt—albeit clumsy and sometimes dangerous—to break through and transcend the limitations of an uninspired and devitalized lifestyle." Since these drugs are criminalized in the West, they find themselves in use often under chaotic conditions that produce confused and nonproductive experiences for the users.

De Rios and Grob in 1992 discussed the role of hallucinogenic plants in adolescent rites of passage in three traditional non-Western societies of the world.[6] In the West, individualism is an undisputed value. Since the end of World War II, the empty self has emerged among the U.S. middle classes, with the breakdown of family, community, and tradition. Alienation, fragmentation, and a sense of confusion and meaninglessness pervade Western society, which particularly affects young people. There is a compulsion to fill up this emptiness, reflected in various ailments of our society: eating disorders, consumers' buying sprees, and the perceived need for mind-altering substances. We see a rapid rise of marijuana use among young people and often there is progression to patterns of multiple drug use and increased consumption of alcohol and tobacco—all of which contribute to greater morbidity and mortality. Mixed with low self-esteem and peer group pressure, substance use among young people is predictable. Chronic substance abuse can subsequently impair cognitive processes, impede development, and increase the risk of lethal behavior. Among tribal societies for which there is information available, it is known that hallucinogens were used ritually to mark the passage from youth to adulthood. The plants were used for their hypersuggestible properties, in order to create a state in which the moral and social values of the tribe would be easier to accept and assimilate. The visions or dreams were subsequently interpreted by the elders of the community in a way that agreed with the specific beliefs and values of the society— which reinforced in the young ideals of society to make them more fit to survive in their culture. In this way, cohesion of the group was achieved as the result of the intoxication experience. As with ayahuasca in the rain forest, tribal societies used rituals of purification prior to initiation rites. Generally, the plant hallucinogens used were not available otherwise, and in this way, they were protected from abuse. They were used ritually at appropriate times, under the control of an elder member of the group or a religious specialist, a shaman.

Mabit is not concerned about any addictive response to ayahuasca, as it is a general rule that powerful psychoactive substances can be consumed in their natural forms without inducing substance dependence. Natural visionary plant substances are almost never addictive in their natural state. According to him, just the opposite. Oral consumption of natural visionary plant substances may actually enhance a person's sensitivity to the alkaloids contained in those plants. Lower doses become the norm and there is not increased tolerance. Carefully structured ceremonies are the model in indigenous rain forest groups. Tribal and mestizo healers also used rigorous fasting and dietary and sexual restrictions essential to enhancing the effects of the ayahuasca and to avoiding negative side effects. The body's digestive system provides a natural defense against an overdose as it responds to the purging and diarrhea-inducing properties of the ayahuasca. This functions as a safety mechanism and works to detoxify the individual. Traditional peoples see the plant as a spiritual ally, not as a recreational diversion. The ceremonies held at night minimize external visual distractions and promote inner visionary experience. Protective spirits are invoked, and the role of music to provoke certain visual patterns is important to guide the ritual taking place in the patient's inner worlds. Mabit uses models derived from psychoanalysis to explain the powerful therapeutic properties of ayahuasca; he explains them in terms of provoking a general amplification of perceptions, an acceleration of mental functions, and the disarming of rational ego defenses. These encourage recovery and transformation of deep subconscious complexes. Not only are visual imageries involved, but the entire perceptual spectrum is engaged, and auditory and olfactory sensations are enhanced. De Rios noted in her research in 1968–1969 that several healers would actually mix the ayahuasca drink with a cheap perfume, locally called Tabu, so that the strong odor of the perfume would rise into the patient's nostrils during the ceremony. This odor activates the olfactory cortex in a very strong way, in the reptilian and mammalian part of the brain, which often floods the individual with past memories.

Initially Mabit worked with several master curanderos in the region and a few patient volunteers. He does not use an abstinence model. Rather, he respects the addict's innate need to experience altered states of consciousness. The program encourages the ritual ingestion of the ayahuasca vine to ensure rapid psychological transformation. A guided psychotherapeutic process is used to encourage residents to deal with deep somatic memories. One of the goals is to deflate ego defenses and to transcend the ego. This encourages the client to reconcile with his or her spiritual nature.

Mabit's wife, Dr. Rosita Giove, is also a physician and a general practitioner in the city, along with her work in the Takiwasi Center. She has collected data about the number of curanderos and midwives (*parteras*) in different communities in the region of San Martín where the clinic is located. She has commented to us that the number of local healers is decreasing to the point that there are communities without any healers at all. However, some of the curanderos travel to different locations. Ayahuasqueros are only found in Tarapoto and other cities; she speculated that the drug tourism is responsible for that. Native healers are not recognized by the government. The lack of dialogue between curanderos and the medical doctors and nurses is fairly widespread. It is clear that no public health policy in this area focuses on the barefoot doctor movement to bring health to the poor and isolated peasantry. Physicians and nurses are sent to rural and out-of-the-way communities straight after their graduation from university, without any real knowledge of the life and customs in the communities they serve. Mabit believes that there is a need to change the laws regarding the recognition of the role of traditional medicine in general, and the usefulness of ayahuasca in mestizo culture in particular.

Mabit believes that traditional treatments for drug addiction are limited, so he turned to spiritual healers, shamans, with resources unknown in the West. Mabit wanted to fuse the rationalism of Western medicine with the traditional practices of spiritual healing in the region. The ayahuasca visions provide users with insight to the underlying causes of their drug addiction. Tarapoto has been in the midst of the coca-producing area and one of the prime consumer areas of cocaine base. Patients typically remain at the center for 9–12 months and avoid contact with relatives during the first three months. The treatment consists of physical detoxification, with the use of purgative plants to cleanse the body. Mabit also looks at emotional cleansing, at which time the patients can take ayahuasca. He uses shamanic chants, icaros, which modify the effects of ayahuasca and provide feelings of peace and courage. In subsequent meetings with psychologists and psychiatrists, the patient is able to interpret the visions he or she had during the ayahuasca session. There are also 10-day retreats in the midst of the jungle, with limited diets, with no electricity, and with nothing to do. Mabit claims a high success rate, stating that over one third of the patients who begin treatment are cured. Among those who complete the treatment, the success rate goes as high as 70 percent. Mabit echoes the work of the psychologist Cushman, that lack of meaning in life is what generally leads to drug addiction, and if society does not deal with this, it will be very hard to eradicate drug addiction.

Mabit's Results

Takiwasi has treated more than 380 patients. A recent study, covering the first seven years of work from 1992–1998, examined drug addicts or alcoholics who completed at least one month of treatment and had been out of the clinic for at least two years. Some 32 percent of patients leave during the first month, before the first ayahuasca session. About 28 percent reached the sixth month of treatment, and 23 percent finished the entire treatment. Two thirds of the patients consumed a highly addictive and debilitating cocaine-based paste. Eighty percent consumed alcohol alone or in addition to other drugs. More than half of the patients had tried other treatments, including psychiatric services. Clients averaged 30 years of age and had been consuming psychoactive substances for about 12 years. Clients tended to pattern into good, better, or same. The first had a favorable development, and their problems apparently were resolved at several levels affecting their lives. The second group showed favorable development with some structural changes, but some of the original problem was still present. The third group relapsed into consuming substances, although they less frequently abandoned the cocaine paste for alcohol use. Findings were 31 percent for the good group, 23 percent for the better, 23 percent were the same or bad, and

23 percent were unknown. Overall, about 62 percent of the patients positively benefited from the model used at the Takiwasi Center. A large percentage returned to Takiwasi if they relapsed, and a quarter of the relapsed patients found other local practitioners of traditional medicine. This demonstrated a high opinion of the approach used at the center. Mabit summarizes the impact of his work as approaching ancient knowledge with respect and careful study. He sees a possibility of reinstating an authentic relationship with the "mystery of life," by validating the legitimate quest of the drug user and then redirecting it to a structured meaningful experience, in order to avoid the extremes of "anything goes" or the useless bellicosity of "everything is forbidden."

*   *   *

Mixed in with the new shamans are remnants of the past, the mestizo healers that de Rios chronicled in her work in the 1960s. Don Tomas from Iquitos is another example of this, as he now works closely with tourists. Eighty-nine years old, he has been working for 60 years. He used to have a tambo (a small enclosure with a thatched roof, open on all four sides) in the rain forest for his apprentices on diets but now only holds curing ceremonies with ayahuasca in Iquitos. He accepts all tourists, who usually come to get rid of their depression, stress, anxiety, or similar psychological problems. He claims that three ceremonies at most are the norm to heal. He also cures children who suffer from daño and digestion problems. In the past, he used to cure adults who suffered daño as well, but now his family does not allow him to do it, because they are afraid that don Tomas will not protect himself enough and will become a victim of the witch's hex responsible for the daño in the first place. With children, the witch does not get involved once the daño is done. Don Tomas always asks the patients about what kind of disease they have and what medication they have been taking. He does not give ayahuasca to the patients with heart problems, psychiatric disorders, or those who have been taking antidepressants or other pharmaceuticals which affect the nervous system. He starts out with a small dose. If the patient does not feel any effect and asks for more, he will give another small dose. Don Tomas is very upset by the charlatans, especially by a woman who calls herself "la diosa del ayahuasca" (the goddess of ayahuasca). He does not recommend a particular curandero to any visitors who want to become an apprentice: he is afraid to send them to a charlatan and then be left to take the blame. In his room, don Tomas has an icon of the Virgin Mary, and sometimes he calls on her for her help during the initial part of the ceremony, to decrease the patient's nausea. He sings icaros in Spanish, but he does not address the saints (unlike, for example, the curanderos in Takiwasi).

Yet another mestizo shaman is don Victor from Iquitos. He is Shipibo, 40 years old, and he has been working for 20 years. He cures with ayahuasca ceremonies, the use of tobacco, and with other plants. Curanderismo is a family tradition. His father, grandfather, and maternal uncle are all curanderos, and presently he is teaching his 14-year-old son to become one too. He works with his uncle and another man in his center, which was recently established. Previously, don Victor worked in his village in the Rio Napo.

Don Victor's center is only for visitors who want to stay for a while and learn about the plants. Visits last at least two weeks long, but some visitors come for a complete apprenticeship, which lasts two years. He emphasizes that it is not a hotel, and he does not accept any tourists. He regrets that there are so many charlatans in Iquitos. Three curanderos teach the visitors in turn: each one works one month long. In this way, the teachings do not conflict with each other. Don Victor holds joint ceremonies with other healers, and he has been thinking about somehow joining several curanderos together to pool their knowledge.

Foreigners come to his center with psychological problems. Most of the local people suffer physical ailments, and until the recent past, there was no medical center available in the Napo region. Don Victor said that in Iquitos everyone suffers from love problems. People come for various kind of pusangas (love magic potions) as well as seeking love, friendship, or success. Occasionally, he has had to work against *hechiceros* (witch doctors). To become a witch, the apprenticeship period only lasts two weeks, instead of two years. Diets of poisonous plants are taken, after which a hechicero gets a virote (thorn) in his throat that forces him to kill people; otherwise he cannot relax. (Others say a virote is a dart that is used by a hechicero to kill someone else, instead of this type of force in the hechicero's body.) Don Victor claims that confidence and faith are very important. He stated: "I could cure you with a glass of water, if you have enough faith." But he explains it as the power of God. Overall he is a devout Catholic. He tells his patients the truth. If he cannot cure them, he simply tells his patient that. For example, he would never admit to curing end-stage cancer, although he says it is possible to do so at the beginning of that illness. However, he thinks that it is very important to give the patients confidence that they will get better. Thus, he thinks it is necessary to talk and joke around, "even though you're crying inside with the patient."

Interviews were held with another two female neo-shamans. The first one, doña Alicia in Iquitos, has a center on a major highway in Iquitos. She is in her mid-sixties, a mestiza who learned from a Shipibo shaman at the age of 16, after he cured her from a lethal disease. Alicia cures with ayahuasca and other plants and uses a different plant from chacruna, chacropanga (unidentified plant), in preparing her ayahuasca drink. Everyone seems to have an opinion about her, ranging from ecstatic approval by tourists to very skeptical comments by other curanderos. Alicia is a really good business-woman, but she did not offer much information in the interview. She indicated that she would share more information if we stayed in her center for at least a few days to take ayahuasca with her, paying cash for everything. She claimed that as a woman, she had to fight against prejudices all her life. Belief has it that a woman cannot cure when she is pregnant or during her menstrual period, and that women cannot learn as well as men. She said this was nonsense. Alicia also claims that all illnesses begin in a person's mind. In addition to the usual depression and anxiety, she says she cures psoriasis and migraine headaches. She believes in "healers from other dimensions" who help her cure patients. Alicia accepts any and all tourists, but she asks them about their diseases and medications first, and she does not give ayahuasca to those who suffer heart disease or who are on antidepressants. She travels around the world to conduct ceremonies as well. She does not believe in witchcraft or the effectiveness of love magic and thinks that it is all superstition. There was a testimonial from an Israeli woman, 23 years old, one of the tourists who visited Alicia. After the first visit she was told that she would absolutely have to take ayahuasca seven times, in about a two-week period, to get rid of her problems (lack of direction in life). She had very strong diarrhea and vomiting in the first ceremony. The second one went only slightly better, and she became unconscious during the entire third ceremony, to the point that, according to the others, Alicia was worried and kept taking her pulse. The woman finally recovered and finished her seven-ceremony cycle with no more fainting but very strong physical effects each time. Two weeks after she left the center she claimed overall satisfaction with her experience and thought that it was interesting and fun, although not exactly illuminating.

A Local Critic of Drug Tourism

A tourist guide whom we will call Ernesto was born in Callao, a port city near Lima. He feels very strongly that drug tourism in the region is a travesty. He dedicates himself to tourist work as a guide. Not only is he a critic of shamanic tourism, but he criticizes tourism in general, throughout Iquitos and the Amazon. When speaking about shamanic tourism that is offered up in hotels and inns in the Amazon, he points out that there is no guarantee for the tourist who decides to ingest the purge, with regard to the quality of the drink she is given. Moreover, no one has qualified the shaman to any standard, and almost always, in his opinion, the whole deal is carried out by people without any experience who are simply contracted by tourism companies. To this, Ernesto adds that the conditions of tourism in Iquitos and the Amazon are deplorable, with few exceptions. Transporting tourists to healing centers can be a dangerous undertaking. There is no authority in Iquitos (the same is true throughout the Amazon) which controls or oversees conditions of the boats that carry tourists outside of the large cities. If they capsize or are run into by other boats, the lives of the tourists are in danger. Moreover, the hotels that lodge the tourists generally are in bad shape, particularly regarding basic amenities such as bathrooms and kitchens. The majority of the 100 or so tourists who arrive daily to Iquitos are victims of tourist agencies who never fulfill what they offer. Particularly, they offer the tourists glimpses of animals like monkeys, crocodiles, anacondas, and jaguars, which is pure hype. The tourist agencies call Iquitos the "ecological capital of the Amazon." However, Iquitos is one of the noisiest cities of the world, because in its streets more than 30,000 motor-cars circulate, producing an infernal noise and contamination. These are altered motorcycles that have a cab attached seating two or three people, making for a bumpy, unprotected ride. By the same token, Iquitos is the city with the least green area per capita in the Amazon. It has less than three square feet of green area per inhabitant, when the acceptable mean is 24 square feet per inhabitant.

In contradiction to its self-proclamation as the ecological capital of the Amazon, in Iquitos we see a great variety of products sold in the markets, especially in the market of Belen. Meat and eggs of species in danger of extinction are everywhere. In tourist restaurants in the city, we see lizard meat, turtle eggs, and other rare items of endangered species. And if this is not bad enough, shops of the city offer a great variety of artisan products made with jaguar and crocodile teeth, as well as guacamayo parrot feathers and those of other birds generally in danger of extinction.

For Señor Ernesto, one of the oldest and best-established tourist guides in the Amazon, the best tourists are those who respect the rule of the traveler, who have interest in nature and who are sparing with the temptations of the tourist market. He finds the best travelers in this respect are the Americans, Australians, Japanese, Dutch, and Finnish. On the other side of the coin, according to him, are the Argentinians, those from Lima, and the Spanish. For Ernesto, ayahuasca tourism is a true risk for the well-being of the Amazon.

As we have seen, new shamans do not think they have a special calling, nor do they heal for moral or providential justification. These attitudes and activities are quite different from the União do Vegetal Church, both in Brazil and the United States, which we will look at next.

CHAPTER 5

THE UNIÃO DO VEGETAL AND THE U.S. SUPREME COURT

In 1961, a new religious group was formed in Brazil, the União do Vegetal (abbreviated here as the UDV); its current membership is over 9,000 people in more than 100 *nucleos,* or communities, one of which is in the United States, in Santa Fe, New Mexico. The plant hallucinogen ayahuasca is used as a sacrament and is ingested at least twice a month in the group's religious rituals and ceremonial events. The sacrament offers spiritual, emotional, and ethical support to those who ingest the tea. As individuals drink, they became part of a religious congregation with the major goal of developing spirituality among members. The tea as used within the UDV ceremonies serves to heighten spiritual understanding and perception, and it is said to bring the religious participant in touch with God. Many who drink the tea participate with their family members present.

Brazilian governmental agencies granted official permission for the ritual and religious use of ayahuasca in 1992; they were influenced by the existence of active ayahuasca-using groups including the UDV and also the Santo Daime, another Brazilian church that uses ayahuasca as a sacrament. In the 1970s and 1980s there was a long-term informal tolerance of such ayahuasca-using groups. As these groups began to expand nationally, however, a campaign was initiated to include ayahuasca (and other plants with which it is combined) on the Controlled Drugs List. DIMED, the governmental agency responsible for the control of production, distribution, and consumption of drugs in Brazil, placed ayahuasca and its additives on the list. After negative reactions from religious groups, an expert commission was appointed. The first one in 1986 reported its conclusions, recommending that the plants be excluded from the Controlled Drugs List. Then in 1987 and 1992 this decision was reconfirmed by two other commissions. Procedures were established to permanently legalize the ritual-religious use of ayahuasca in Brazil.

Ayahuasca as a Sacrament in the UDV

Baker[1] has written about the use of psychedelics as religious sacraments. Many who use ayahuasca have argued that the use of psychedelic substances in a religious context, in order to provide spiritual insight, has been a part of human history over millennia. The example most often cited is the supposed use of Kykeon as part of Greek religious rituals connected with ancient Eleusian religious rituals. While the term "sacrament" usually brings to mind Christian rituals, specifically, the seven sacraments of the Roman Catholic Church, the term can be used in conjunction with new religions such as the UDV. Some recognized usages of the word "sacrament" that are pertinent to our discussion include that of a pledge of a covenant between God and man, and the concept of making sacred or consecrated. Many drug tourists, for example, believe that ayahuasca helps to reveal an aspect of divinity within themselves, the self-spirituality to be discussed shortly, as they advance on a vaguely defined spiritual path. One supposes that tens of millions of individuals since the 1960s have explored psychedelic substances to access their inner worlds, and certainly some may have obtained important religious and spiritual insights. Much of this exploration, however, has been idiosyncratic and not experienced ritually within an established cultural tradition. Generally, with drug tourism there has been a lack of specific beliefs and practices surrounding the use of these substances in the West. Nor has there been culturally codified dogma set up in a way that shapes the drug intoxication of participants even before they have these experiences. Most idiosyncratic users do not have an interpretive framework to use once they ingest ayahuasca. An old adage from the 1960s says that if drugs are used ritually, little abuse follows.

In this sense the UDV, while not standing alone, is one of the few organizations that currently exists to help individuals interpret the ayahuasca experience within a specific religious symbology. Motivations of drug tourists for using ayahuasca clearly differ from those of UDV members. Such motivations of the drug tourists can range from mere curiosity to a sense of adventure to a desire for spiritual insights. The concept of religiosity in a sociological framework—dating back to Durkheim[2] and earlier—looks at the cohesiveness of a group. This is clearly minimal or absent among the drug tourists when compared to the UDV members.

The ayahuasca that is grown and harvested for the UDV rituals is prepared by church members according to standardized recipes that vary only slightly in their *preparo* (preparation) ceremonies. Other psychoactive substances like marijuana or cocaine are rejected by church dogma. There is supervision by and vigilance of adepts during the ceremony. Experiences are interpreted within the explanatory framework of Christian and spiritist doctrine understood by the leaders and church members. Moreover, the church has had great success in helping members recover from addiction to alcohol and from cocaine abuse,[3] to be discussed shortly.

The Organization of the UDV Church

The UDV is a Christian spiritist organization set up with a hierarchic structure that is composed of a Master Board, a Council Board, an Instructive Board, and a Member Board. As with many spiritist and spiritualist groups throughout Latin America, followers are arranged according to their level of spiritual development, called "degree," as well as by their service to the organization. Oral transmission of beliefs has played an important role in the church. The shared ritual experience of ingesting ayahuasca, or hoasca, as it is known in Portuguese, serves as a teaching vehicle for the followers. The UDV has always maintained a mutually respectful and cooperative relationship with the Brazilian authorities, and it is sometimes called upon to consult with Brazilian authorities regarding ayahuasca's sacramental use there.

Church acceptance today of this plant contrasts dramatically with how other visionary plants were viewed by the European explorers and missionaries as trafficking with the devil. No published evidence exists in any ethnohistorical sources that we have found to show that Europeans took ayahuasca in the early centuries of contact. On the contrary, missionaries throughout Latin America attempted to repress traditional religious beliefs and practices and to "save" the souls of native peoples, by obliging them to abandon their customary practices and to embrace the Christian faith. Over the centuries, as various Christian denominations spread throughout Latin America, syncretic movements arose. This term "syncretism" describes the mixing and blending of the sociocultural components of religious systems. Certainly, over time, religious systems change. Indigenous beliefs and practices have blended with those of the dominant Christian culture, as the result of conquest and domination by Europeans. All over the world, Christian beliefs have been assimilated into traditional indigenous cosmologies to become powerful symbolic images and rituals. Roman Catholicism in particular has blended with pagan traditions in the Americas. Add to this mix slaves imported from Africa to Latin America and the Caribbean, who brought with them traditional religious ideas and practices that were also combined with Roman Catholicism. Some of these religious sects include Umbanda, Macumba, and Candomblé in Brazil. Syncretic traditions grew up that combined traditional African religions, Kardecism (spiritism), and Catholicism. The influence of Kardecism, discussed earlier, is very important in the UDV Church.

The UDV is one such syncretic religion. It tends to be apolitical in nature and devotes itself to maintaining a spiritual role in contemporary Brazilian society. It does draw upon shamanism, the religion of the hunters and gatherers, which values an altered state of consciousness as the means to control and dominate spirit forces in nature. In shamanic-based societies of the world, numerous individuals have access to such altered states of consciousness, as well as the perception and awareness of the spirit world. The hoasca tea enables UDV members to achieve a state of consciousness akin to this shamanic experience. The art of curing, a major aspect of shamanism, plays a much lesser role in the UDV rituals, however.

UDV members believe that the use of hoasca as a sacrament permits them to develop their spiritual lives and to contact the spirit world. From this experience, an individual is believed to be able to receive knowledge, power, and well-being. There are important Christian elements, as well as beliefs from mestizo culture. The "Lord's Prayer," occasional signs of the cross, and a strong preoccupation with charity and moral rectitude are the Christian elements that are incorporated into the UDV tenets. Unlike many other Brazilian religions, the UDV does not favor dancing or maraca drum beats as part of its ceremonies.

A Description of UDV Ceremonies

De Rios visited 11 UDV temples in four cities of Brazil—Sao Paolo, Rio de Janeiro, Brasilia, and Manaus—and interviewed numerous members of the church. Approximately 70–80—members and visitors were present at each of two hoasca sessions she attended in 1999. The UDV temples were large, with bright electrical lights and a photograph of the founder, Mestre Gabriel, which hung prominently on a wall. The major activities of members of the religious community were to clean the premises, to prepare food for the evening activities, to garden, and to maintain the temple. Child care was available to permit adults to attend their activities during the day, the evening meal, and the ceremonies. The ritual took place in the evening, about 9:30 p.m. The officiating *mestre* (religious elder) asked for the attention of the members who were seated around a central table with individuals of high rank. The rest of the participants were seated on comfortable chairs along the walls of the temple. The core group of mestres and counselors stood up and in silence recited a short prayer to themselves. Then, each member in the temple was served a glass of the hoasca tea; this was done quietly and in an orderly manner. The mestres and counselors drank first and in a larger amount than newcomers. Before taking the tea, the participants prayed individually and gave thanks. During the initial half hour when the hoasca was taking effect, the rules and statutes of the UDV were read. Most of the participants wore a green shirt with the UDV emblem. No one drank alcohol or smoked during the sessions. This half-hour period ended with a prayer or *chamada* to Mestre Caiano (Cain, in the Old Testament), asking that he guide the ritual toward the path of light.

When the tea began to take effect, some participants had to leave to vomit or go to the bathroom, as the purgative properties of the tea were felt; individuals periodically stood up and asked permission to leave once these purgative effects made a bathroom visit necessary. They returned quietly to their seats afterwards. The mestre asked individuals how they were feeling and if they were experiencing the effects of the *burracheira,* or consciousness change. During the next two hours, the tea had its maximum effect, and more prayers were recited. The Portuguese phrase "luz y força" (light and force) were spoken frequently. There were lengthy periods of silence when most of the participants were concentrating in silent meditation and paid little attention to others around them. Many kept their eyes closed. Occasionally, soft recorded music with a pronounced beat was played. During the sessions that de Rios attended, she heard sermonizing from the officiating mestre, who insisted on the necessity of leading a correct life and seeking the light. There were group discussions of moral and theological issues and brief testimonies of various ones' personal illumination. Recreational drugs were denigrated and considered vices. Those with such habits were said to be "lost ones."

There was a general euphoria produced at the end of the ceremony, as people believed they shared a common perception of a transcendental reality. Four or five hours after taking the drink, the mestre asked the group: "how was the burracheira?" All answered "bem" (meaning "well" or "excellent"). A final oration was recited, and an appeal was made to Mestre Caiano. The session was formally closed at that time. Outside the temple, hot tea was served, and small groups congregated as in any social reunion after church services. Many talked about their visions in the session. Afterwards, people were genial and interactive and appeared genuinely pleased with their experiences. From the point of view of antianxiety effects of the hoasca, the tea appeared to help people feel connected to one another and to a common cause—their church.

Some adolescents were present and took part in the ritual. De Rios did not see them experience any adverse reactions to the hoasca tea. She attributed the absence of adverse effects to the fact that the mestres interviewed potential visitors who wanted to take the hoasca tea prior to the ceremony.

In this way, individuals they deemed to be unstable would not be permitted to drink the tea.

On one occasion, in a Sao Paolo temple, de Rios saw a young man stand up and, in a rigid posture, assume several combative martial arts poses. The counselors seated at the main table were aware of his behavior and occasionally inquired as to his well-being. She was later informed that the youth had a history of drug abuse. He was said to be seeing scenes of his past unfold in his visions. However, this was without any of the screaming or writhing in horror de Rios had on occasion observed during bad trips among ayahuasca takers in the Peruvian Amazon in the late 1960s, when she attended sessions there. De Rios was impressed by the strong value system of family and community that she observed among individual members of the UDV Church. While there were some single-parent families and single individuals, the overwhelming majority of people were part of intact nuclear families, and adults and children alike were actively engaged in church activities. De Rios observed two young teenage boys crying because for one reason or another they were not able to attend a UDV session one evening. It certainly appeared that the UDV church provides an integrative experience for its members that is neighborly, community-based, supportive, and spiritually satisfying.

Hoasca and Redemption

De Rios conducted a formal interview in a Manaus temple with 10 mestres of the UDV Church. Individuals reported that their lives had been changed for the better. The UDV has literally hundreds of stories of men and women who formerly abused alcohol, cocaine, or heroin and who had violent and unproductive lives before they became involved with the church. The concept of redemption and personal change was cited by de Rios' informants as being the result of their hoasca experiences and their identification with and involvement in church life and activities.

The UDV Adolescent Study[4]

In the late 1990s a study was designed by researchers from the United States and Brazil to examine the effects of ayahuasca on a group of Brazilian youth, ages 12–19, who had been given the sacramental hoasca tea since they were in their mothers' wombs. Since their birth, they had drunk the tea on a regular basis. Unusual in such drug research was the use of a control group composed of other teens who had never taken ayahuasca but who were matched in terms of age, gender, socioeconomic status, and level of education. None of the youth in the control group were members of the UDV.

The control and experimental groups were recruited from the local high school population in the cities of Sao Paolo, Campinas, and Brasilia, Brazil.

The UDV youth had taken ayahuasca twice a month as part of the ritual activities connected to their church. The concern of the Brazilian government was that this powerful hallucinogen might create learning and adjustment problems for the teens. Overall, the findings showed that there was no significant difference between the two groups on any of the test measures. The tests examined speeded attention, visual searching, sequencing, psychomotor speed, verbal and visual abilities, memory, and mental flexibility. Statistical data were computed on both the UDV teens and their counterparts in the community. It is very hard for the anthropologist in a fieldwork situation—in the tropical rain forest, for example—to set up what scientists call a "bench study," where all the variables to be studied are carefully controlled. The cooperation of the UDV church was instrumental in allowing our binational research team to successfully undertake such a study.

To our knowledge, there are no other studies such as this which give conclusive results about the effects of powerful hallucinogens used in a ritual setting. In personal conversations with some of the UDV adolescents, de Rios noted that there was a certain concern expressed that some of the teens' friends thought they used ayahuasca just to "get high," when the youth involved held the sacrament in great respect and awe for its spiritual value in their lives.

Focus groups conducted by a sociologist were held in all three areas of Brazil. They were tape-recorded and transcribed for analysis. The youth were questioned on their prior history of alcohol, marijuana, cocaine, and amphetamine use. A general history was taken as well.

Certainly, in Western society, giving drugs to children brings up visions of evil and sinister wrongdoing, action worthy of an immediate call to child abuse registries for their prompt investigative and punitive action. The cooperation of the UDV in enabling this study to occur gave the researchers a rare opportunity to study the world-perception, social values, and the beliefs of some 80 adolescents with regard to similarities and differences between the two groups. Formal neuropsychological testing in Portuguese was conducted in both groups, along with interviews held and questionnaires answered, to learn more about how these youth were getting along in life.

Mostly, when we think about drug-induced consciousness among young people, we have visions of alienated, introspective, rebellious boys and girls. All sorts of illegal behaviors come to mind. For the teens in the UDV church, however, we see ritual and ceremony surrounding the drinking of the tea, a sacrament that gives spiritual, emotional, and ethical support to those who drink it. The young people join in with their religious congregation and, through this religious event, are expected to develop spiritually.

A number of interesting findings give us insight into the UDV as a social organization and into its influence on members, both youth and adults. The UDV adolescents were just as involved and responsible as the controls. The UDV teens always reported chores they had to do, compared to the controls, who often had maids at home to do the work. More of the UDV teens reported living with both parents compared to control teens. The quality of home life was examined, and it appears that the UDV teens have a better quality of home life when compared to their peers. The UDV teens also appear to have a closer relationship with their fathers compared to the controls. UDV teens overwhelmingly drew their friends from church members and relied less on friendships with schoolmates, compared to control teens. The teens were hesitant to discuss their religious practices with schoolmates, who simply assumed that they were only involved in the drug aspect of religion to get high. The concepts of societal alienation and integration within the society were also examined. The UDV teens differed in the perception of violence and corruption in society, and the UDV teens were more optimistic than their peers.

Five vignettes were designed to function as neutral stimuli, to tell a story that revolved around a moral dilemma. Each youth was asked to complete the story—for example, they were to answer a question such as "what would you do if you saw a classmate stealing money from your teacher's purse?" When moral and ethical values were queried, there was a significant difference between UDV teens and controls. The UDV teens showed stronger loyalty to family and friends. When asked about formal religious affiliation, there was a significant difference between UDV teens and controls regarding religious practices. The control group was overwhelmingly Roman Catholic. Of the UDV group, six also belonged to spiritist temples. The five vignettes were developed to measure moral and ethical considerations of both the UDV and control teens. In modern-day industrial societies, drug and alcohol use is often associated with excessive risk taking, impulsivity, and, at times, a disregard for safety and consequences. It was believed that the vignettes would permit honest self-reportings by the teens about their potential responses to conflictual situations as well as their general levels of maturity.

Differences appeared in the area of confrontation, and it appeared that controls were more likely to take an aggressive stand when confronted. The UDV teens, like the controls, found clandestine premarital sex to be distasteful. The UDV teens were realistic in not wishing to be antisocial and offend their parents. This could be interpreted as a mature recognition of the importance of family in third world societies, both economically and socially. The young people who participated in the ayahuasca religious ceremonies, usually with parents and other family members, appeared not to differ significantly from their non-ayahuasca-using peers. Few, if any, differences in responses between the UDV teens and the controls were found. The UDV group seemed to be more responsible, respectful, and concerned about the welfare of others. They exhibited greater optimism than their peers. They valued virginity before marriage and avoidance of drugs (other than ayahuasca used sacramentally).

We might expect that, given the destructive consequences of youthful drug use in contemporary Western society, that the UDV teens would lag far behind their peers in a number of different dimensions of sociability, honesty, studiousness, and other such character traits. In fact, it would be easy to assume at the outset of such a study as this that the UDV teens and the controls would differ in some significant fashion. However, the qualitative data reveal that the UDV teens appear to be healthy, thoughtful, considerate, and bonded to their families and religious peers.

The U.S. Supreme Court and Ayahuasca in the United States[5]

A recent decision of the U.S. Supreme Court (2006) has legalized the use of ayahuasca in the U.S. branch of the UDV Church. Known formally as the Centro Espirita Beneficente União Do Vegetal, the church has received numerous civic awards and governmental recognitions of distinction in Brazil. Also recognized as a church under the laws of the United States, the UDV Church's members drink the ayahuasca tea within their religious services. Members believe that the tea heightens the individual's spiritual understanding and perception and brings religious practitioners in touch with God.

When U.S. Customs inspectors confiscated 30 kilograms of the UDV's ayahuasca tea in New Mexico, the tea had been prepared in Manaus, Brazil and shipped to the United States. The UDV was threatened with prosecution. The government argued that the DMT (dimethyltryptamine) in the additive plant can cause psychotic reactions, cardiac irregularities, and adverse drug interactions. The UDV cited studies showing that its sacramental use of hoasca was safe. The lawsuit brought by the church sought tolerance and accommodation of its practice of receiving communion using the ayahuasca tea—a practice that it argued was central and essential to its faith. Representatives of the United States government previously threatened to arrest and prosecute members of the UDV if they continued to practice their religion in the United States. The UDV argued that it was only seeking the rights it believed are guaranteed under the First Amendment to the U.S. Constitution and under international treaties and domestic law. The latter is primarily based on the Religious Freedom Restoration Act of 1993 (RFRA).

Under this 1993 legislation, the main causes of action within this federal law are intended to protect the free exercise of religion, and to provides access to the courts for sincere individuals and recognized churches who are not able to exercise their religion freely because of actions by the federal government. The U.S. government defendants in this case conceded that the UDV is a recognized religion, that its members are sincere, and that the government's actions prevented UDV members from practicing their religion. Once such a situation arises and the religious group challenges the government's prohibition in court, the RFRA requires the government to prove to a federal judge that it has a "compelling interest" that can only be served by banning a particular exercise of religion. This means that the government has to show that the religious conduct in question, if allowed, will cause serious harm.

The government defendants claimed that hoasca was dangerous to the health of the UDV's members, that the UDV's hoasca was likely to be diverted to nonreligious use, and that permitting the UDV's members to import hoasca from Brazil would cause the United States to violate an international treaty. After two weeks of testimony, including that given by eminent experts in the fields of medicine, drug control, and law enforcement, the district court judge ruled that the government had failed to prove it had any compelling interest at all. The government failed to show any health danger, any likelihood of diversion, or that if the UDV were permitted to import its sacramental hoasca it would cause the United States to violate any treaty.

The government conceded that it failed to prove a compelling interest in prohibiting the UDV's religious use of hoasca. It then argued that the district court should have found that the government's burden was satisfied merely because hoasca contains a very small amount of a Schedule I controlled substance, DMT. The possession and use of DMT is against the law. This argument by the government, if accepted, would have effectively repealed the RFRA. This is so because the RFRA's only role is to address conflicts between federal laws and the free exercise of religion. Whenever such a conflict arises, the RFRA requires that the government must prove why it is so important that a particular law be applied to prevent a particular religious practice. But in the case of the UDV, the government took the position that it should not have to prove anything more than to show that the UDV's sacramental hoasca contains a very small amount of a controlled substance. Therefore, the UDV was violating the law. In other words, having failed to prove that UDV's exercise of its religion is harmful to anyone, the government then took the position that it should not be required to prove anything at all. The government's position has been correctly perceived by religious groups in this country to represent a serious attack on the RFRA itself. If the government had been successful, it would have made the RFRA meaningless and put in jeopardy other religions' exercise of their rituals.

The RFRA had been passed into law in 1993 by unanimous voice vote in the House of Representatives and by a vote of 97–3 in the Senate. Constitutional scholars and elected officials from both sides of the aisle considered it to be one of the most popular and important laws Congress has passed in recent history. In a case before the Supreme Court earlier in 2005 related to the "establishment of religion," that court noted that it had not yet ruled on the constitutionality of the RFRA as it relates to federal law. However, neither party in this case questioned the constitutionality of the RFRA. Thus its constitutionality was not an issue before the court. The question arises whether the outcome of this lawsuit has been important only to UDV members or whether it has wider implications.

We need to understand some of the constitutional principles involved in the long legal battle the UDV had with the U.S. government.[6] The U.S. Constitution's First Amendment leads us to believe that the writers of this document were concerned with controlling the elites' power—represented by the state—and this can be applied to the right to oversee other people's consciousness. This derived, no doubt, from centuries of religious-based oppression and political domination in Europe. When dispute and divergence arose, it intended to establish circumstantial "accommodation." The First Amendment does not allow the federal government to promulgate any law that pertains to establishing a religion or prohibiting free exercise of such a religion.

Some Pressing Issues

Before the U.S. Supreme Court rendered its decision about the legality of the UDV's use of ayahuasca as a sacrament, Dr. de Rios and Dr. Grob interviewed the UDV's chief mestre here in the United States, Jeffrey Bronfman, about his thoughts on the case (2005). He spearheaded the legal battle to allow his church to partake of the ayahuasca tea used sacramentally in its Holy Communion.

Bronfman had been working for a number of years with a private foundation that funded environmental conservation and the preservation of tribal cultural traditions. During that time, a proposal crossed his desk from a spiritual organization in Brazil that wanted to preserve an certain area, because of the numbers of plants central to their religious practice that were growing in abundance there.

Through his studies and travel, Bronfman was already aware of the long history of psychoactive plant decoctions used among indigenous societies in magical and religious rites. Initially, he traveled to Brazil to investigate this environmental conservation project, as well as to learn more about this religious tradition that used indigenous Brazilian Amazon plants ceremonially, as a sacrament.

Bronfman spoke about the growth of the organization today to have more than 10,000 members throughout Brazil and in the United States and Spain. Each congregation normally has from 75 to 200 adherents, who receive Holy Communion through the ingestion of the tea at regularly scheduled occasions (approximately two times per month).

When asked to describe any similarities between the UDV and the Santo Daime movement (to be discussed shortly), Bronfman said that the founders of both religions encountered the sacramental use of the tea while working in the deep interior of the rain forest as rubber tappers. Both later went on to establish different sects, where the tea was to be used in ritual form for the purpose of communion with God and the elevation of the spirit. Neither originator of the UDV or of the Santo Daime knew each other personally, but they did know of each other's work, and each held the other in high esteem.

Bronfman discussed how the UDV became legally established in the United States in May 1993 and set up its bylaws. The church submitted an application for recognition to the Department of the Treasury, which through the Internal Revenue Service supervises the licensing of all nonprofit organizations. When the tea was confiscated in May 1999, the organization became involved in a very demanding legal controversy with the Drug Enforcement Administration (DEA) as well as the Department of Justice regarding its sacramental use of hoasca. The DEA and the justice department took the position that the UDV's religious use of the central sacrament of their faith is prohibited under domestic drug laws. The church took the position that its practice is protected under the laws that guarantee the free exercise of religion. When the DEA seized the shipment of ayahuasca, the UDV negotiated for 18 months to try to get the sacramental tea returned. The UDV believed that this seizure was a failure to respect its most basic human right—to freely exercise its religious practices—and that the DEA was neglecting its own sworn duty to uphold the U.S. Constitution. This prompted the church's decision to take the offending agencies to court. Documentation and legal arguments for both sides were presented to the federal district court, and at the end of October and November 2000, there was a two-week hearing on the case. The UDV waited nine months to learn the outcome and received a favorable decision from the court. The UDV was granted a preliminary injunction in its favor, protecting its religious practice and the sacramental use of the hoasca tea from interference or threats of criminal prosecution by any agency of the U.S. government.

The UDV spent several additional months negotiating an agreement to implement this order with representatives of the Department of Justice and the DEA, when the defendants appealed the district court's decision to the 10th Circuit Court of Appeals before the ruling could even go into effect. The case was heard by a three-judge panel from the appeals court. After nine months of deliberation, there was a divided two-to-one decision that granted their preliminary injunction. The decision affirmed the district court's decision; they agreed with the lower court's judgment that the defendants' actions were in violation of federal laws that protect free religious exercise.

In the judgment of the majority, the defendants had not met the burden assigned to them by Congress under the law. Government agencies cannot interfere with, or prohibit constitutionally-guaranteed freedoms. Again, before this second judgment and order could take effect, the justice department, the DEA, and the U.S. Customs Service once again appealed. They asked for a rehearing of the case by all of the active judges of that court. Their request was granted in January 2004. Oral arguments were presented before a 13-judge panel in March 2004. As we will see shortly, the eventual hearing of the case before the U.S. Supreme Court ended favorably for the UDV.

Bronfman believes that what was at stake in this case is a principle of freedom so fundamental that it is hard to imagine its denial in the United States. This country was conceived with notions of liberty and freedom of religious expression, and it was hard for the mestre to even speculate about a negative outcome for the UDV.

*   *   *

The outcome certainly is of essential importance to Congress, as well as to the religious and civil rights communities. This case determines whether the courts will apply the RFRA as Congress wrote it or not. If the government had been correct that it could satisfy its burden under the RFRA merely by proving that something is against the law, then the RFRA would have been rendered meaningless. This is because the RFRA's protections are only triggered when a particular exercise of religion violates a law or regulation. So in order to win its case the government said it needed only show that the UDV's exercise of religion violated a law. Then the RFRA would not protect anyone's exercise of religion.

The U.S. Department of Justice asserted that hoasca was illegal under the Controlled Substances Act. The UDV responded that the RFRA, as passed by Congress, applies to "every federal law," including the Controlled Substances Act. As a religious sacrament central and essential to the UDV religion, the use of hoasca is not prohibited under the Controlled Substance Act unless the justice department could have proven (through evidence) that it had a compelling interest in applying the act to the UDV's religious use of hoasca, as well as that there is no "less restrictive" means of meeting that interest as it relates to the 140 U.S. UDV members. Two federal courts in three opinions said the government had not provided such proof.

The justice department also asserted that hoasca was illegal under the 1971 Convention on Psychotropic Substances, and that the U.S. government was obliged to adhere to this treaty. The UDV's response was that the government's responsibility under any international treaty can never be used to justify the denial of a constitutional right, or violation of a domestic law such as the RFRA. The treaty in question was effectively amended with the passage of the RFRA, which was written after the United States signed and ratified the treaty. By its terms, the RFRA applies to all existing federal law. The Official Commentary to the 1971 Convention (which is the equivalent of its legislative history in explaining the treaty's intent) states that the treaty does not apply to plants and infusions made from plants. It also speaks specifically of "toleration" of the use of "plants growing wild which contain psychotropic substances from among those in Schedule I, and which are traditionally used by certain small, clearly determined groups in magical or religious rights." Furthermore, the 1971 Convention contains a provision that excuses compliance if its application in a particular context would violate a country's laws or constitution, as is the case here since both lower courts have found that the government's refusal to accommodate the UDV's religion violates the RFRA.

Many people have wondered how the UDV's situation compares with that of the Native American Church and its legal use of peyote. The UDV legal counsel argued that the government's accommodation of the Native American Church clearly demonstrated that the federal government could easily accommodate the UDV's religious practice without undermining the nation's drug laws. Interestingly, some have argued that the supreme court has made ethnocentric assumptions by placing peyote at Schedule I status, since it is recognized as safe and therapeutic.[7] The membership of the U.S. branch of the UDV is about 140 people, while the number of members of the Native American Church is estimated to be 250,000. Within the Native American Church there has been no evidence of a diversion of peyote among those who sacramentally drink a tea containing peyote or chew the cactus in religious ceremonies.[8] In fact, Chief Justice Roberts of the U.S. Supreme Court wrote that "if peyote was permitted...for hundreds of thousands of Native Americans practicing their faith it is difficult to see how those same findings alone can preclude any consideration of a similar exception for the 140 or so American members of the UDV who want to practice theirs."[9]

The evidence submitted to the court showed that the similarities between the UDV and the Native American Church are truly remarkable. Both are modern expressions of religious traditions using plant material as a form of sacramental communion. Their origins go back hundreds of years. The two churches, both of which are Christian in theology, were organized within 80 years of one another, in both cases predating the current controlled substances laws. The government has readily agreed that the Native American Church's use of peyote, also a Schedule I controlled substance, has caused no health or drug problems in this country. The government has never been able to convincingly explain why the UDV's use of hoasca should be seen as dangerous.

The justice department asserted that if the UDV was allowed to use hoasca for religious purposes, the plant would then easily have been diverted into the general population and become a drug of abuse. Once again, the evidence does not support these assertions. The UDV imported hoasca for more than 11 years without any diversion from its use as a religious sacrament. Under the injunction imposed by the federal district court and the current license from the DEA, the UDV has, since December of 2005, resumed the importation of hoasca for its religious services. No diversion has occurred. Furthermore, there was extensive expert testimony to establish that the nature of hoasca is such that it would be a very unlikely candidate for a drug of abuse, given the strong emetic effects commonly experienced. Now that the UDV has prevailed in its lawsuit, a question arises: can anyone in the United States use hoasca, or can only UDV members use it?

The answer is that the federal court's decision relates only to the religious use of hoasca within the "clearly defined, circumscribed context" of the UDV. Is this a slippery slope? Since the UDV has prevailed in this case, can we say that this will open the door to the legal use of hallucinogens? Hallucinogenic substances, in general, remain illegal under federal and most state laws. The accommodation that is being granted to the UDV is based upon the organization's legitimacy, the history of its religious use of hoasca, and the absence of evidence that it is harmful or that it would be diverted to illegal use. Another group wishing to utilize a psychoactive substance central to its religious practice would have to be prepared to prove its case in court, if the government maintained that it had a compelling interest in prohibiting the use of that substance. The accommodations for religious use under the RFRA do not extend to "recreational use," as the district court and appeals court opinions have made very clear. Adherents of the UDV are certain that there is no "slippery slope."

Analysis

There is an interesting conflict in the way that information about ayahuasca is presented by the UDV compared with the government's presentation. To paraphrase an old brief written on behalf of Timothy Leary in the 1960s, "to examine the beliefs of one religion is to examine the beliefs of all religions." While the government calls ayahuasca mixed with DMT a drug, the religious users call it a sacrament. Its transportation from the site of preparation to the church where it will be used in worshipping rituals is called traffic. Its effects, recognized by adepts as divinatory, therapeutic, or oracular, are regarded by the government as hallucinatory, risky, and harmful to one's health. The U.S. Supreme Court justices gave this case very serious consideration and took a very cautious and skeptical position when confronted with superficial arguments lacking evidence. They compared this case with the historically controversial case regarding the use of peyote in a ritual-religious setting within the Native American Church. Certainly the battle is far from over. New twists and turns in UDV use could be returned to the lower courts. For now, the respect for religiosity that characterizes Brazilian society has made its mark on American jurisprudence.

Chief Justice Roberts wrote that the government had not demonstrated a compelling need. The law required the government to consider on a case-by-case basis whether its action could infringe on the freedom of religion. Other religious groups such as the Baptist Joint Committee said the decision was good news for religious freedom and the fact that the Religious Freedom Restoration Act continued to be a vital force in American life.

Santo Daime

Another ayahuasca church found throughout Brazil and also abroad is the Santo Daime Church. The name does not honor a saint but is translated as a form of prayer to God, with "Santo" meaning "holy"; it asks for health, peace, and other attributes of a spiritual life in the command form of the verb "to give." The Santo Daime Church is a syncretic group that incorporates indigenous practices of ayahuasca use with elements of Christianity. It was founded in the 1920s by an unusually tall African-Brazilian rubber tapper, named Raimundo Irineu Serra, who lived in the state of Acre. He was influenced both by Catholicism, prevalent since the sixteenth century, and spiritism, prevalent in Brazil since the end of the nineteenth century. Under the influence of ayahuasca, Serra had a vision of the Queen of the Forest, a white woman dressed in blue whom he believed to be the Virgin Mary. Through his visions, he was instructed to found a new religion with ayahuasca as the main sacrament. Concepts of reincarnation, salvation, and protection of the rain forest characterize the beliefs of this group. The Queen of the Forest is worshipped as a teacher, and the ayahuasca tea is used for enlightenment and healing. In this church, the use of hoasca permits the development of spiritual life as well as contact with the spiritual world, which provides knowledge, power, and well-being. In addition to ayahuasca, the church also uses cannabis (marijuana) as a sacrament. Daimista centers have been established throughout urban areas all over the country since the early 1980s, and today Santo Daime groups exist in Europe, Asia, and North America.[10]

Early in its history the church gained followers among other rubber tappers, then it spread to poor rural Brazilians in the town of Rio Branco. After the decline of the rubber boom, many of the rubber tappers were forced to migrate to the cities of the region, where they faced great difficulties integrating into urban society. As the church splintered into several smaller groups at the death of the founder, one branch became very active, attracting foreigners and middle class adepts.[11] It reached major urban areas in the state of Acre. With harassment by the Catholic Church, Santo Daime headquarters were moved to a village called Ceu do Mapia (heaven of Mapia) in 1981. The governing body is a Spiritual Council in the Ceu de Mapia rain forest preserve; this council makes policy decisions. Some Brazilian celebrities journeyed to Ceu do Mapia, bringing publicity to the group, and over the years other churches have been founded in major metropolitan centers including Brasilia. Today, there are several thousand adherents worldwide. The clergy consists of spiritual leaders known as Padrinhos and Madrinhas who act as guides, but the plant is said to be the true teacher. Their scripture utilizes the Catholic Bible as well as the writings of Mestre Irineu, the founder, which are mainly in the form of hymns. These writings are called the Third Testament of the Bible. Before taking the hoasca, the ritual participants are asked to refrain from eating red meat and dairy or having sexual activity. As a syncretic religion, the Daime revere Jesus and Christian saints as well as African and indigenous deities.

Preaching in the church is carried out by a collective performance of hymns and a synchronized dance called a *bailado*. The dance is accompanied by vigorous percussion and the playing of melodic instruments. All participants are required to sing and dance during the ceremonies, which can last from 4–12 hours. Barbosa and his colleagues examined first-time ayahuasca users, among both the Santo Daime group and the UDV in Sao Paolo and Campinas, Brazil. Individuals were asked to help map the altered state induced by ayahuasca and were interviewed about their lives and physical and psychological well-being. Although the numbers of people interviewed were small (19 among the Santo Daime and 9 among the UDV), the results are worth examining. This was a highly educated sample of people in both groups. Most were sensitive to the supposed properties of ayahuasca as a medium of spiritual or psychological development and improved health. The Brazilian urban middle class appears to have a high regard to seeking spiritual and mystical experiences, as an alternative way of life to the growing materialism and utilitarian values developed in recent years in Brazilian society.[12] There is what Barbosa[13] calls "a 'prevalence of metaphysical religiosity' that incorporates practices and beliefs accompanying alterations of consciousness." Clearly New Age movements have made inroads in Brazil, and beliefs in reincarnation contribute to the positive and optimistic attitudes of these subjects toward their ayahuasca experiences. Barbosa points out that insights experienced during the altered states are crucial to self-knowledge and spiritual evolution. Barbosa's studies indicate that it is possible that the UDV participants were more stable emotionally than those in the Santo Daime group. Perhaps, as that author points out, the lack of singing and dancing are responsible for this.

The Brazilian federal government has shown concern that the Santo Daime sect was duping people and robbing money from its members. A Federal Drug Council investigated the group in the 1980s and released a report that the use of ayahuasca posed no danger, but rather it had a positive, beneficial impact on the group's communities and on social integration. The church is established in the United States, Japan, Holland, and Portugal and its membership was augmented by New Age seekers. In Brazil, many of the followers come from a background other than that of rural mestizo farmers or indigenous peoples. Many have a secondary or university educational level, and members suffer from personal problems and psychological issues. Brazil today has large-scale unemployment, inflation, and the near-disappearance of what was a relatively prosperous middle class. Culture changes and the breakdown of the traditional family and its values are everywhere. Groups like Santo Daime provide many with a sense of their own identity from a social, psychological, and spiritual perspective.[14]

Brazil had been one of the few countries officially permitting the use of the ayahuasca vine for religious purposes. With the recent U.S. Supreme

Court decision to allow the União do Vegetal Church to use ayahuasca and *Psychotropia viridis* as a religious sacrament, ayahuasca has been accepted as part and parcel of at least two new religions. The tropical woody vine is fairly difficult to grow in nonequatorial climates, except in greenhouses. Thus the UDV in the United States continues to import the tea from Brazil. At the 1992 Earth Summit, Ceu do Mapia became the center of a million-acre ecological preserve, purchased with the help of Friends of the Amazon. Efforts are under way to create an international center in Mapia to offer workshops in traditional healing, ecology, and consciousness studies. It is currently estimated that between the two ayahuasca churches there are 10,000 to 20,000 Brazilians who participate in ayahuasca-based religions. The number of followers who live abroad is uncertain.

Ayahuasca visions among Santo Daime ayahuasca tea drinkers include visions of the Virgin Mary as Queen of the Forest and of Christ. Additionally, great importance is attached to the Milky Way as a road of the dead and a veridical link between the cosmos and the earth. Santo Daime sect members have reported visions of flying through or above the galaxy in space and meeting aliens who claim to originate from the galaxy's center.

When the founder of Santo Daime, Irineu Serra, or Mestre Irineu, died in 1971, there were several factions in the church. One called CEFLURISS has been central in the subsequent growth of the church. Like the UDV, it attracts middle-class Brazilians and visitors from abroad who want to partake of its rituals. Chapters have grown in a number of urban and rural centers, as well as overseas. As Tupper has relayed, there have been a number of legal actions against the church in the Netherlands, Spain, and Italy. In Canada, in the province of Quebec, the church applied for an exemption to the Canadian Controlled Drugs and Substances Act to try to avoid a legal battle. There is an interesting conflict between churches trying to legitimize the use of the ayahuasca tea as a religious sacrament and liberal democratic states endeavoring to uphold religious freedom while at the same time retaining punitive drug laws.

Brazilian Cultures of the Amazon

The Santo Daime Church hardly exists in a vacuum. In addition to having an uneducated rural population of rubber tappers and gold miners in the Amazon region, religions in Brazil have been influenced by African spiritual beliefs. There is a large black and mixed-race population, with Brazilian race relations professing equality for all ethnicities in the country. Yet clear segregation exists in the professions and the military.

An important influence of European spiritism dates back to the nineteenth century, when mediums in the United States increased in number and spiritualist churches in Brazil were established. Séances and belief in reincarnation and spirit contact have been widespread through Brazil. Mesmer's influence and his concepts of animal magnetism and theosophy spread to Brazil from European immigrant influence. Also influential was Kardecism, discussed earlier.

There is a class- and race-based stratification within the religious structure of Brazil. Dark-skinned mestizo groups have tended to seek out the syncretic folk religions. Some people from the lighter-skinned upper classes have shown interest as well. These Brazilian new religions include Umbanda, Candomblé, and Macumba. They share some traits with the Voudoun and Santería religions of the Caribbean. However, Santo Daime and the UDV differ from these other syncretic religions in their use of the ayahuasca tea. This compares to the use of trance possession and other altered states in these Caribbean religions, states which are induced by drumming, meditation, and chanting. To some, ayahuasca acts as a bridge between the Amazon forest and its cities, bringing together Whites, Afro-Brazilians, native Americans, and mestizos.

CHAPTER 6

GLOBALIZATION AND THE FUTURE OF AYAHUASCA

The future of ayahuasca is inevitably linked to the populist movement in the United States. This is especially so because of the free and open access of the internet for those interested in ingesting the hallucinogenic tea, whether at home, in the Amazon, or abroad. Many believe that plant psychedelics are innocuous and free from danger. Marijuana, ecstasy, psilocybin, and others all fall into this category.

Thomas L. Friedman[1] defines globalization in a way applicable to the drug tourism we are looking at. He sees globalization as having "its own demographic pattern—a rapid acceleration of the movement of people from rural areas and agricultural lifestyles more intimately linked with global fashion, food, markets and entertainment trends." We saw in Chapter 2 how many of the mestizo ayahuasca healers have moved to cities, leaving few healing resources in the outback areas of the rain forest. Runaway drug use in American society is now giving rise to the demand for more entertainment for international travelers, with ayahuasca sessions mixed in with mud bath rituals and other bizarre techniques. Individuals in this model are super-empowered; they do not need to be part of any political setting but can act directly on the world stage.

Zealots for drug use are very pleased to see increased research being published to fortify the medical use of these substances. A nonprofit organization, the Multidisciplinary Association of Psychedelic Studies (MAPS), has spearheaded a movement to permit research with a variety of these psychedelics, generally within a medical or harm reduction model.[2] The organization has worked with skeptical federal authorities to win necessary permissions to grow some plants such as marijuana for research purposes, and to have them available for research with human subjects. Marijuana policy reform lobbying is growing in support. Major science journals like the *Archives of General Psychiatry* and the *Journal of Clinical Psychiatry* have published articles that show clear benefits in the use of psychedelics to treat mental illness. Certainly there are innumerable anecdotal reports about the anxiety-reducing effects of ayahuasca. Mood and anxiety disorder research at the National Institute of Mental Health found "robust and rapid antidepressant effects" that continued for a week with depressed subjects who were given ketamine. Core obsessive-compulsive symptoms were reduced for most patients when given psilocybin in a controlled medical setting. Those published studies, needless to say, urge caution, and the researchers generally see the utilization of these treatments happening only after all other pharmacological and psychological interventions have failed.

It is possible that psilocybin may facilitate psychological insights and help to reduce psychiatric symptoms in low doses. It may even provide profound existential and spiritual realizations to about 30 percent of those who take the substance. Nonetheless there are contraindications which in a clinical setting in the United States would not be tolerated. For example, any individual who is vulnerable to psychoses, severe mental disorders, would be at risk. Anyone with overvalued ideas—obsessions—or who exhibited violence toward herself or others would need to be carefully screened.

The Future of Ayahuasca: Medical and Psychological Aspects

Medical potentialities of ayahuasca are only beginning to be examined. As early as 1927, a renowned German drug researcher, Lewin, conducted experiments with ayahuasca in the psychiatric clinic of the University of Heidelberg. When ayahuasca was given to patients suffering from encephalitis, muscle stiffness completely disappeared. Another German scholar, Beringer, gave some of the alkaloid to patients suffering from Parkinson's disease and observed stiffness and gait improvement.[3]

When psychedelics are used in European and American societies, and when its use is illegal and seen by many to be antisocial, the experience will be structured by the values and knowledge of the individual. Such a person will most likely be critical of some laws such as those prohibiting psychedelics and be likely to identify with a subculture and not the society at large. As the individual user is open to suggestion during the acute phase of the psychedelic ingestion, she may be receptive to ideas and values that counter traditional Western values. In the West, these substances are defined as drugs of abuse. Since few people die from overdoses of the psychedelics, the individuals taking them are not likely to appreciate the values of their society which proscribe their ingestion. Thus these plant hallucinogens are prohibited by society and fly in the face of established cultural values. This often leads individuals to distance themselves from the group and to lack any sense of group cohesion. Individuals, thus, reject the most basic ontological assumptions of their society.

After more than 35 years of restriction regarding research on psychedelics, there is a growing number of studies that look for ways to treat intractable mental illness with hallucinogens. Such subtances include ecstasy, marijuana, psilocybin, and even ayahuasca. Some promising studies show that medical applications of psilocybin for obsessive-compulsive disorder facilitate psychological insights, and, at very low doses, reduce symptoms.[4] The substance is well tolerated by volunteers, who reported a decrease of their symptoms and had profound personal and spiritual benefits from the experience. Like all studies for the last 40 years or more, pre-drug screening is important. Individuals who are likely to develop psychoses or severe mental illnesses are not candidates for psilocybin. Those who have overvalued ideas, what the French call "une idée fixe," also are kept from participating. Of course, those who show violence toward themselves or others are definitely not appropriate subjects. After the sessions, the individuals need careful debriefing, and they should be treated by competent and supportive individuals. Psilocybin has been seen as useful in the treatment of post-traumatic stress disorder and depressive diseases that are resistant to the standard list of antidepressive medications. Recent studies by Grob utilize psilocybin for anxiety experienced by cancer patients in advanced stages of the disease. Some researchers show interest in using drugs like MDMA (ecstasy), which cause less altered sensory perceptions compared to LSD. This can be used with patients who have not been successful with traditional therapies. From an existential perspective, these substances are said to create very powerful religious and spiritual insights for the individual and to unlock repressed feelings. The MDMA is said to enable patients to enjoy life and make productive contributions. There is a large anecdotal history lauding this substance's positive effects in facilitating psychotherapy.

Finally, peyote has long been used by Native Americans to treat illness. As de Rios and colleagues found, there is a redemptive element to the use of some of these psychedelics in helping individuals abstain from alcohol, heroin, and other drugs of abuse. The downside is that many of these herbal psychedelics like peyote and even ayahuasca may, within a generation or so, become endangered species, chewed or drunk up and no longer sustainable.

These psychedelics need to be subjected to scientific scrutiny and experimental control before passing into general psychiatric use.[5] Their toxicity levels have to be established as well as their safety and effectiveness.

Drug Tourism: The Netherlands' Free-for-All

Drug rituals using ayahuasca have caught on in the Netherlands. Participants who want to drink ayahuasca are attracted by means of advertising in shops, by direct mail, and by word of mouth. In the late 1990s, ayahuasca use became popular in this area. In 1993, the first ayahuasca rituals were held in Amsterdam, organized by Santo Daime church members. Elements of Roman Catholic, African, and Amazonian beliefs were characteristic of these activities. The brew was brought from Ceu do Mapia, Brazil. Men and women were segregated, they used different uniforms for different ceremonies, and periods of both reflection and dancing rituals occurred. Hymns were sung from the Santo Daime's Third Testament. In addition to the Santo Daime rituals, a mestizo curandero, originally from Iquitos, performed ayahuasca rituals at this event in Amsterdam. He blew tobacco smoke into the ayahuasca brew as his clients watched. Whistling is believed to evoke the spirits of the plants, and the tobacco smoke eliminates any negative energies of people. The curandero also used chacapa leaves to provide a drumming-like sound to accompany the ingestion of the tea. Arno Adelaars,[6] writing in a European journal, described rituals conducted without any religious structure, given the general disenchantment of many Dutch people with Christian religious symbols, along with their low church attendance. Ayahuasca has moved into a more recreational context. The plant and some of its additives have become available to the European market and a "do it yourself" (DIY) ritual is currently widespread. Ad hoc guides come to the scene to help their friends throughout an evening of drug taking that is reminiscent of the 1960s in the United States and elsewhere.

Cultural Appropriation[7]

Anthropologists get very upset at the way that powerful nation states, both historically and in the recent past, have appropriated indigenous knowledge and even spiritual wisdom. The fifteenth century Spanish conquest of Latin America is a good example of this. Syncretism, or blending of doctrines and beliefs of many major religions with native deities and rituals, has been well documented by anthropologists and historians. The Europeans and Americans systematically sought to assimilate native peoples into colonized territories and to destroy their traditions. De Rios wrote about French colonial policy, for example, which as late as the 1950s tried to impose a "civilizing mission" to alter the basic structure of West African societies under their political control. Some anthropologists consider this to be a form of genocide, or at the least, discrimination and racism. Even the plant ayahuasca has been patented as if it were an invention and not a member of the plant kingdom!

The appropriation of ayahuasca and its rituals, and even the rise of White Shamans, as they are called—Westerners pushing aside indigenous or mestizo healers to take over their rituals—is referred to as biopiracy.[8] The empty self discussed earlier needs to be filled up with calories, drugs, sex, and power, and the ayahuasca user is a sitting duck! As we saw in the discussion in Chapter 3 on drug tourism, local authorities have been unable to organize the ayahuasca healers in any meaningful way to set some minimum standard of care and screening before dispensing ayahuasca to strangers. The modern saga of powerful chemicals and food and medicine interactions can only bode badly for the future of ayahuasca.

Rituals or No Rituals with Ayahuasca

This concept of DIY—"do it yourself"—with ayahuasca is surely the wave of the future, given the belief of users in the power of the plant to provide them with insight and psychological relief from distress and anxiety. Anthropologists have a long history of analysis of rituals in society since they appear to meet specific needs of human beings. David Smith, the founder of the Free Clinic Movement in the United States, and de Rios[9] examined the function of drug rituals in human societies. They found that despite a long history of drug use in hunting and gathering societies, among early agriculturalists and in early state-level societies, rituals, rather than DIY sessions, were the general rule. In fact, ritualization of drug ingestion is one of the near-universals that anthropologists encounter.

When we look at societies historically, before the rise of the state, we find that in lieu of legal restrictions on use, ritual has controlled the powerful effects of drugs. When such rituals exist, problems of abuse are minimal. The rituals that surround the use of a drug historically function to prevent untoward effects. Such ritual would include how the drug was procured and administered, what settings were selected for use, and what activities occurred after the drug was given. Social norms were in place in these societies that determined how or whether a particular drug should be used, including informal and often unspoken values or rules of conduct shared by a given group.

With the frontier mentality in American history, the growth of self-reliance and individualism is given lip-service in European-American societies. There is a carryover to drug use with substances like ayahuasca. Rituals in human society have served many purposes and generally are established for prescribed procedures of a ceremonial or formal act. In traditional societies of the world, drug use occurs within the context of sacred meaning, when people recognize a more-than-human realm that has to be dealt with in a customary way. Beliefs and rituals go together and cannot be separated. The belief that is connected to the drug use explains, rationalizes, and directs the energy of the ritual performance. "Do-it-yourselfers" believe that psychedelics are therapeutically necessary for their spiritual health. An expanded consciousness is said to put a person in touch with universal energies and to confer positive benefits on his spiritual health.

We have seen the role of redemption through ayahuasca use among members of the UDV in Chapter 5. In societies of the world where a person's self-esteem is low and human beings experience negative emotions such as fear, despair, emotional disorganization, and crises of personal identity, psychedelics, along with other substances like alcohol and tobacco, have functioned to help individuals attain renewal. This can be seen in the Native American Church's use of peyote, as Native Americans face cultural disorganization. It can also be seen in other nativistic movements, such as the Bwiti Cult in West Africa, where the psychedelic Iboga is used by the Fang people in rituals to ameliorate the effects of a century of French colonial control.[10] Yet another way to look at the DIY approach, or recreational use of psychedelics, is to observe how individuals let off steam, in what anthropologists call "rituals of rebellion." People are required or allowed to do the wrong thing, so that order and stability in society can be maintained. Rituals of rebellion allow impulses to be vented that otherwise would be chronically frustrated. Normally when we speak about rituals in society, we find that they promote the social solidarity of a group, a concept well illustrated by the UDV Church. Rituals bring people together in situations where quarreling is forbidden.

American society lacks socially accepted models for controlled use of psychoactive substances. The use of psychoactive drugs carries criminal penalties, and criminal justice procedures rather than rituals regulate and control their use. To avoid such criminal treatment in the United States because of ingesting psychedelics, more and more interested parties are finding their way to Peruvian, Brazilian, Ecuadorian, and Venezuela rain forests to taste the merchandise. And that is indeed what ayahuasca use has become—more and more a DIY endeavor and tricksters' merchandise.

The Changing Shaman

In a book on shamanism published in Germany in 1999, the psychologist Stan Krippner listed the primary characteristics of successful shamanic healers. Among the characteristics that Krippner viewed as essential for successful healing were 1) a shared world view that provides meaning to the diagnosis given; 2) personal qualities of the practitioners that facilitate the client's recovery; 3) positive client expectations such as hope, faith, and placebo effects to assist healing; and 4) a sense of mastery on the part of the client that creates empowerment. If we apply these characteristics to the new shamans discussed in this book, we see some real problems. First of all, many of the clients speak little if any Spanish, and most of the shamans stumble by in basic "the-bathroom-is-down-the-hall" kind of English. Sterling members of the community they so often are not, as we saw with ones who rush to drug their client, recently arrived by plane from Lima or other major cities, or who negotiate high fees for the ayahuasca session; many do not have the slightest idea about how the body functions. Certainly with regard to faith, hope, and placebo effect, most clients come with recommendations by friends and acquaintances who have had interesting experiences, so their expectations are generally high. The fourth characteristic generally means that experienced practitioners of other hallucinogens—which description characterizes many of the clients—are relatively easily able to endure the ayahuasca trip, despite the purging effects. This is certainly a long way from either indigenous or mestizo healing discussed in this book.

Ayahuasca and Globalization

If we look at globalization as increased ease of movement for ideas, goods, and people, as the twenty-first century unfolds we see changing political, cultural, technological, and economic transactions occurring. These, in turn, affect our understanding of psychedelic substances such as ayahuasca and the meanings the plant has for different groups of people. These groups include the native Amazonian residents, indigenous, rural, or urban, as well as middle-class men and women from Amazonian countries like Brazil, Peru, Bolivia, Ecuador, and Venezuela. Additionally, foreign tourists come to seek the plant as a medicine, teacher, or a spiritual advisor. Colonialism and imperialism change their form, but they certainly do not disappear. Appropriation of native use of this plant hallucinogen appears to be inevitable, as the drug tourism described in Chapter 3 indicates. Perhaps this conundrum will disappear as the continuing touristic influx causes the plant species to disappear and become extinct. Certainly ayahuasca has fallen off the plant list of numerous indigenous Amazonian groups who now practice tobacco shamanism, given their lack of access to viable and sustainable ayahuasca sources. Trends show that the future will continue to include commercialization and secularization of ayahuasca.[11] In this age of the internet and file sharing, indigenous peoples' use of ayahuasca will hardly remain protected or kept out of plain view. The term "commodity" here means any product or service available, and it brings the question of who can provide the ayahuasca service cheaper. Women, too, are becoming ayahuasca healers, despite the recent past prohibition of allowing menstruating women to participate in healing rituals with ayahuasca. The authors interviewed three women healers who did not even seem to remember the clear constraints on their presence in—let alone mentoring of—the ayahuasca sessions not so long ago. During 1968–1969 when de Rios worked in Iquitos, although she interviewed 12 ayahuasca healers, none of them were women. Only one older woman, past menopause, accompanied a healer as he sang his icaros. Women who were involved in witchcraft activities were much more common, preparing love potions for their clients to bewitch jealous rivals or make their lovers impotent with other women. Let them conduct an ayahuasca session?—no way.

Right now, prices for ayahuasca sessions appear to be rising, but there are more and more ayahuasca providers springing up daily. Profit margins will surely diminish, and as competitors increase, there will be a tendency to sell more, do more web pages, and have more agents abroad—or lose business!

As we have seen in Chapter 5, the spread of ayahuasca rituals by a number of religious groups, not only in Brazil but in Europe, the United States, and Canada, has resulted in legal challenges to the use of this plant as a sacrament. From the position of a "drug," a "psychedelic," or a vice, the plant has been reframed by some as a medicine, a sacrament, or even a plant teacher.

Legal challenges to the use of ayahuasca throughout the world have occurred in Australia, Italy, the Netherlands, and Spain. Plants like ayahuasca do not fall easily into categories of drugs of abuse, along with the medical marijuana lobby, or the psilocybin seen by Grob to ease suffering and death anxiety for end-stage cancer patients. The policy expert Tupper argues that there is a question we must think twice about, what he calls a deficit model of drug use that focuses squarely on harm reduction. In his evaluation, policy should be reframed to look at benefit maximization.[12]

Historically, ayahuasca has been condemned by colonial and religious authorities as "the devil's work," and its use has been widely discouraged. Christian syncretism has added to the mix. An example from de Rios' fieldwork is interesting to observe here, as she observed a Peruvian coastal ritual in 1967 with the mescaline cactus San Pedro. The healer, when offering a mescaline drink to patients who had come from far away to imbibe the San Pedro infusion, made all the gestures of a Roman Catholic priest that de Rios had observed the prior day at a funeral mass in the local Catholic church. Psychedelic plants have been cast out of their traditional frame and are now part of the worldwide tourist movement.

To date there are no real longitudinal studies of ayahuasca on continuing drinkers. Anecdotal accounts, however, are commonplace. Grob's 1994 UDV study[13] found that not only was there no physiological or psychological harm discernible when ayahuasca was used in ceremonial contexts, but in fact, there could be said to be redemption at work among individuals who previously were addicted to heroin and cocaine. Many had led lives of violence and desperation before becoming involved with the UDV Church.

Among a group of 15 ayahuasca-using individuals who reported a variety of dysfunctional behaviors before their entry into the church, 11 had a history of moderate to severe alcohol use, and five reported episodes of binge drinking associated with violent behavior. Two had been jailed due to their violence. Four of the subjects abused other drugs including cocaine and amphetamines. Eight of them were addicted to nicotine. Many described themselves as impulsive, disrespectful, angry, aggressive, oppositional, rebellious, irresponsible, alienated, and unsuccessful. Eleven of the 15 told Grob that the ritual use of hoasca had a profound impact on the course of their lives, and, while under the effects of the psychedelic, they saw their self-destructive path leading to their ruin and even demise unless they radically changed their personal conduct and orientation. A commonly reported vision was that the founder of the UDV, Mestre Gabriel, would appear and deliver them from the terror they were experiencing. Once involved with the UDV, they gave up alcohol, cigarettes, and other drugs and were careful with their words, practiced good deeds, and developed a respect for nature. There was a profound sense of meaning and coherence in their lives. De Rios found this same pattern to hold among the 11 mestres of the UDV church in Manaus that she interviewed in 1997.

This redemptive concept is often referred to as drug substitution, when one substance is used to obviate and negate the cravings for and withdrawal effects of a second. Methadone is the best-known example. Hallucinogens like ayahuasca that do not cause physical dependence have taken on this function for a number of UDV members who were addicted to other substances such as cocaine, heroin, and alcohol. Ayahuasca appears to have helped bring about more effective psychosocial functioning, and it has helped individuals to assess and alter their destructive patterns of behavior and to avoid using those substance which caused them harm in the first place. Looking at this as a redemptive approach posits that the proper use of one substance can help to free a person from the adverse effects of an addiction to another substance.

As with members of the UDV, this can restore an individual to be a fully functioning part of his or her community or group.

Many writers have suggested that the states produced by hallucinogens can have profoundly positive, even life-changing effects upon individuals. This often happens because they provide insights into meaning and psychological dilemmas. Viewed from a broader cross-cultural perspective, redemption can be seen as a process that entails freeing someone or something from a less-than-desirable state and restoring them to a desired state. There is a change of status that is in the best interests of the person or persons involved.

Since the era of the 1930s in Brazil, the traditional rural agrarian economy has been steadily replaced by an urban, technologically oriented, industrial one This has caused massive dislocation and the migrations of large numbers of unemployed rural persons to urban centers, in search of jobs. Urban life has severely weakened large extended family systems. Given this sociocultural transformation, stress has become widespread as individuals attempt to cope with new and disruptive problems in their environment. Drug abuse has become rampant in large Brazilian cities like Manaus, Sao Paolo, Rio de Janeiro, and elsewhere. This historic period has also witnessed a rise in new religions such as the UDV, as well as the growth and proliferation of older ones, such as the Umbanda and Candomblé, to help individuals solve their personal difficulties. The UDV and its use of ayahuasca can be seen as one attempt to restore personal, familial, and social stability in a rapidly changing world.

Other psychedelics have in recent years been used as redemptive drug substitution, with mixed results. One of the better-known ones is Iboga, historically used by the Fang peoples of West Africa as part of a syncretic ancestor-worship religion. Used in Bwiti ceremonies in Gabon and the Cameroons in high dosages, some fatalities have been reported by anthropologists. The use of the drug is symbolically described as "cracking the skull." This plant has been integrated into Western clinics in the Caribbean and Vancouver, British Columbia; it gives rise to lucid visions and the emergence of repressed memories. There have been a number of clinical reports on the essential loss of opiate craving and the absence of withdrawal for several months in the literature on drug substitution. Overall, the plant visibly alleviates morbidity and appears to remove addicted individuals' desires to seek and use narcotics.

In particular, one of the global themes connected to hallucinogenic use that was first discussed by de Rios in 1984 is that of a sense of death and subsequent rebirth, which allows the user to return to a new beginning.

The physical effects of vomiting also provide a sense of cleanliness and individual renewal. The suggestibility properties of these substances can be managed by a healer or shaman to achieve psychological goals and cognitive restructuring—rethinking tired and nonproductive ways of organizing information and behaving.

Even LSD, in its early years of use in the 1960s, generated a large scientific literature on the application of this psychedelic to effectively treat alcoholics. Both a continuing low-dose experience and a one-time high- dose experience were used with clients, designed to loosen or dissolve tensions and conflicts within the psyche. It was argued that these mind-loosening sessions made it possible for patients to work through and resolve the material responsible for their alcoholism in a rapid fashion. In the altered state induced by LSD, a religious experience would then be created. Patients were encouraged to reassess their beliefs, the ways in which they interacted with others, and their value systems. Those addicts who had a transcendent response to LSD were far more likely to demonstrate a sustained improvement in their overall condition and to remain abstinent. As de Rios pointed out in 2002, whether the drug substitution is done in a secular context through a medical model or in a religious context such as with the UDV, sobriety for that addictive drug which caused disequilibrium to the individual in his or her social context is the ultimate goal.

Perhaps, as Winkelman argues,[14] hallucinogens are "psycho-integrator plants with therapeutic benefit."[15] Since these substances have sensory, behavioral, emotional, and cognitive effects, they integrate not only the mind, but also the soul and spirit. These substances alter experience by shifting awareness to an experiential domain that the individual interprets as sacred.

Ayahuasca and Abrupt Global Warming

The Amazon basin is the land of water. Coursing through an area of 18 million square kilometers, the Amazon River encompasses more than one quarter of the world's currents of water and 20 percent of available drinking water in the planet. The volume of Amazonian rivers represents almost half of the sum of all water movement on the earth. The river is 6,780 kilometers long and is the largest in the world. All these waters are changing drastically and abruptly for many reasons, especially as the result of global warming and its immediate consequences. Temperatures are rising from the Atlantic and Pacific tropics, provoking inclement droughts. Water levels in Iquitos have reached their lowest level in 35 years. Forest fires have covered the sky with smoke in practically all of the Amazon basin, and navigation in the affluents of the Amazon has been at a point of collapse due to lower water levels.

In the city of Acre in Brazil, no rain fell for four months in 2005, and the rivers dried up. In Mato Gross, Rondonia, and Maranhao, Brazil, there were some 40,000 forest fires over a five-day period. A dense smoke covered the streets and penetrated the houses in Rio Branco, Cruceiro do Sul, and other cities of Brazil, with hospitals declaring an emergency, concerned over general asphyxiation. These changes can be catastrophic for the entire chain of life that the Amazon River sustains and feeds, especially for human life.

It is interesting to note that the pre-Colombian indigenous population of the region was estimated to be between 7–10 million inhabitants. Today it is estimated that this population, after 500 years of colonization, is 1,500,000 inhabitants, in some 13 ethnolinguistic families. Many of these peoples have used ayahuasca in their religious rituals for millennia, and many continue to do so today. These tribal groups have well adapted over thousands of years to the rain forest. Their world views are animistic and pantheistic, and for them, nature is sacred. This contrasts dramatically with the world view of the West, where nature and its reality are fundamentally materialistic. The indigenous tribesman or woman is attuned to the world of nature, the Amazonian plants, minerals, and animals. Shamanism was the glue that linked the different realities together. These beliefs have influenced the urban Western culture today in the Amazon. We can only imagine how these climatic changes will affect the growth and availability of ayahuasca—as well as cause destruction, population changes, and massive cultural change in the not-so-distant future.

This concept of major changes taking place in the Amazon forest is seen to be inevitable. In Brazil, as we will see shortly, there is a very rational approach to dealing with the forest, with many enlightened laws set up to protect the environment and to regulate ayahuasca use. However, many writers see these laws as "paper tigers" having no enforcement due to lack of funds. Brazil is unable to monitor or enforce these laws on the books in protected areas. As mentioned, fires are burning out of control in the Amazon basin, destroying millions of acres. In 1987, an area larger than Switzerland burned in less than a month. These large-scale changes affect not only Amazon countries such as Brazil, Peru, Bolivia, or Ecuador—but the world as well. Economic development in the area, including logging, mining, and agriculture, all leads to massive forest loss. The rural populations are becoming urbanized. Just as governments are unable or unwilling to manage the excesses of drug tourism, they are also unable to manage the destruction of the environment.

The Rational Voice of the Brazilian Government[16]

In November 2006, the Brazilian Anti-Drug Council (CONAD) published a position paper on ayahuasca that gives us an excellent blueprint for the future. In this document, the government of Brazil regulates religious/sacramental use of the ayahuasca tea. The working group within the organization was composed of representatives of the religious organizations that use the tea, as well as jurists, anthropologists, public health and public policy experts, and physicians. Recommendations of this working group were accepted by council and now are government policy in that country. Focusing on *Banisteriopsis caapi* and *Psychotropia viridis,* the two major components of the ayahuasca tea, the group recognized ayahuasca as protected by the Brazilian state, **within a ritual setting.** Religious groups properly registered with and recognized by the state can cultivate and prepare ayahuasca for their own consumption. There is a focus on the importance of making the plant self-sustainable, that is, cultivating the plant so as not to see it become an endangered species, with each religious entity working to achieve this goal. Brazil's federal constitution guarantees free exercise of religious organizations.

The recommendations negated internet offers of obtaining the plant, any promises of miraculous cures, or statements that ayahuasca is a remedy for all illnesses. It distinguishes between legitimate religious use and those practices that are not legitimate, practices outside of religious rituals. There is a focus on allowable use for scientific research and a clear statement ruling against the recreational use of ayahuasca. Touristic information as propaganda of the effects of ayahuasca is discouraged. If a religious group is formally organized, has legal status, and is responsible for its acts, with social projects delineated and having a congregation of coreligionists, it is deemed acceptable for the tea to be used as a sacrament.

The commission was very clear on the avoidance of use by people who have had previous mental disturbances or previous emotional problems. Traditional folk healing was also prohibited (especially because of new information about foods and medicines' harmful interaction with the plant). Moreover, those individuals taking ayahuasca should not be under the effects of alcohol or other psychoactive substances. Prior to the initial drinking of ayahuasca, the individual should be informed of all conditions that exist with regard to ayahuasca use and any potential hazards.

The commission took issue against any commercial uses, ayahuasca in any form being sold for payment. Nor did the group approve of touristic explorations of the tea. Nonritual use of ayahuasca was also interdicted. The commission also saw a need for scientific studies of the therapeutic benefits of the plant. They went on record as being against traditional healing that can put individuals at risk for their mental and physical well-being. Their conclusions were that ritual-religious use of ayahuasca has been recognized as a legitimate practice, both in traditional Amazonian populations and in part by urban populations. The state of Brazil guarantees the right of cultural expression protected by law in the federal constitution.

Each religious group should exercise rigorous control concerning the entry of new adepts. People should be interviewed and screened before they are given ayahuasca. Finally, the commission recommended further scientific studies in the area of pharmacology, biochemistry, clinical psychology, anthropology, and sociology with a multidisciplinary focus. Of great interest was the recommendation that CONAD should promote and finance studies about the effects of ayahuasca, starting in 2007.

Constructivism

Culture is continually emerging and in-process in all of social life. Information on the drug tourism documented in this book is based on our observations and interviews of healers and patients and health and science professionals in the Amazon community. These tourist productions of ayahuasca sessions are systems in themselves. As Bruner points out, there are many different players who have to be studied for their presentation, and not for what they are assumed to represent—such as traditional shamanic healers. Authenticity is irrelevant, as culture is continually changing and becoming reformulated. The tourist performances, even those that take place within the individual's psyche after she ingests the hallucinogen, become part of a new culture which is modified to fit the touristic master narrative. The psychic performances are edited by the healers and are easy for the visitor to understand. Moreover, they take place on a regular basis. Most of the ayahuasca clients interviewed by de Rios in 1968–1969 and in 1977 took ayahuasca with the healer only one time. Our interviews show multiple sessions, often within a week or two, with the client's tolerance for the ayahuasca not held as particularly important. The tourist leaves his home to experience something totally new, and by golly, he had better have the experience, even if it means repeating the performance again and again until he gets it right. Those providing the performance also are creating something new. The postmodern approach to drug tourism would be to see all culture as continually invented and reinvented. The copy is better than the original, and perhaps this is true with ayahuasca tourism. Instead of feeling the fear of malevolent kinsmen or neighbors who wish to bewitch you and kill you and your children, or to cause you to have continual bad luck, the drug tourist wants alleviation from depression, resolution of trauma, achievement of a sense of identity, and other psychological outcomes. Or, perhaps he just wants to get high and have a good time. Whatever is simulated is better, more real, than the original. Ayahuasca use has changed in the last century, these neo-shamans would argue, and why should it not continue to change and reformulate itself? If the interest is expressed mostly by foreigners, so be it, they say.

Conclusion

We can predict that the ongoing globalization of ayahuasca will take one of several different paths in the future. The plant can continue to be abused by charlatans who extract cash from unwary men and women—those hungering for spiritual experiences or psychological help for personal problems. The Peruvian, Brazilian, and Ecuadorian governments should consider a travel advisory in several languages to alert tourists to the potential of charlatanry as they are accosted on the streets of downtown Iquitos or Manaus, or at airports while they wait, with offers of ayahuasca "rituals." Or, the plant can be absorbed and integrated into an enlightened medical/spiritual model, where a cost-benefit analysis carefully evaluates the ingestion of the plant with health and mental health risks. Or the plant will simply be used up and tourists will go elsewhere to meet their needs and fantasies.

Shall we see these substances as malevolent agents and pathogens? Or, are they tools, as Winkelman and Tupper argue? Are they inherently dangerous, or does their alteration of consciousness provide some kind of potential benefit? Are we seeing a replay of the 1960s, when a serious medical lobby saw great potential in the use of LSD to treat intractable mental illness and alcoholism—while at the same time, the intoxicated, LSD-using daughter of a famous television personality jumped off a building to her death, believing she could fly? Using a metaphor of hallucinogen as tool, rather than malevolent agent and pathogen, any plan for future incorporation of ayahuasca into a medical model would come attached with a set of protocols. Such protocols should include the following: bona fides regarding the source of the plant; set and setting control; a mindful sitter of safety; no involvement in risky activities; screening out takers of those with psychiatric disorders; careful diet intake prior to ingestion to eliminate foods containing chemicals that prevent the action of ayahuasca from occurring, and the avoidance of certain substances like antidepressive medications. Any formal use of ayahuasca would entail some kind of screening of practitioners. This unfortunately reminds us of the many pseudoscientific certification boards that spring up like mushrooms after a rainfall in medicine and psychology, where, for a very high fee, one can be a member of a select group of specialists who supposedly meet a minimum standard of competence. This is a problem when, as Arrévalo stated to

Rumrrill in an interview, almost every Shipibo house in Pucallpa, Peru has a resident shaman, now that the profit for offering the experience is so high. In earlier times, there might have been one or two specialist shamans in the community who were highly regarded. Apprenticeships have almost disappeared in recent years, as the commercialization of the ayahuasca rituals has pushed out the traditional knowledge base.

In this book we have looked at the fascinating plant ayahuasca and its potential for good, as well as its dangers. We see the trajectory of its use in ancient shamanic religions of the Amazonian rain forest, the changes among indigenous South American shamans, the usurpation of ayahuasca by mestizo rural and urban river-edge peasant farmers, its incorporation into several new Brazilian religions, and its entry into religious sacraments in the United States. Finally, we see its impact on drug tourism and its European augury for do-it-yourself use. Quite a profile for a simple woody vine, threading its way through the moist tropics of the Amazon.

ENDNOTES

Chapter 1 Introduction

1. Bianchi & Samorini, "Plants," 1997.
2. Halpern & Pope, "Internet," 2001.

Chapter 2 Native Use of Ayahuasca

1. Rodd, "Piaroa sorcery," 2006.
2. Ibid.
3. Siskind, "Visions and cures," 1973.
4. Coppens & David-Cato, "El yopo," 1971.
5. Riba et al., "Effects of South American," 2004.
6. Dobkin de Rios, *Visionary vine,* 1984.
7. Sklerov et al., "Fatal intoxication," 2005.
8. Reko, *Magische,* 1949.
9. Stephens, "Cannabis," 1999.
10. Dobkin de Rios & Janiger, *LSD,* 2003.
11. Gehricke et al., "Smoking," 2007.
12. Dobkin de Rios, *Visionary vine,* 1984.
13. Dobkin de Rios, *Amazon healer,* 1992.
14. Skinner, *Beyond freedom,* 1971.
15. Tart, *Altered,* 1969.
16. Owen-Kostelnik et al., "Testimony," 2006.
17. Eysenck, *Encyclopedia,* 1975.
18. Dobkin de Rios, "Vidente," 1984.
19. Simon, "Mechanism," 1990.
20. Dobkin de Rios & Grob, "Hallucinogens, suggestibility," 1994.
21. Baker, "Psychedelic sacraments," 2005.
22. Dobkin de Rios, "Shamanism and ontology," 1999.
23. Dobkin de Rios, *Amazon healer,* 1992.
24. Dobkin de Rios, *Visionary vine,* 1984.
25. Dobkin de Rios, *Amazon healer,* 1992.

26. Ibid.
27. Dobkin de Rios, "Saladera," 1981.
28. Dobkin de Rios, *Amazon healer,* 1992.
29. Dobkin de Rios, "Fortune's malice," 1969.
30. Dobkin de Rios & Rumrrill, "Interview," 2005.
31. Ibid.
32. Dobkin de Rios, "Vidente," 1984.
33. Tournon, "La merma," 2002.
34. Ibid.
35. Lathrap, *Upper Amazon,* 1979.

Chapter 3 Drug Tourism

1. Dobkin de Rios, "Drug tourism," 1994.
2. Seguin, *Folklore psychiatry,* 1974.
3. Ortega y Gasset, *Revolt,* 1992.
4. Baker, "Psychedelic sacraments," 2005.
5. Dobkin de Rios, "Drug tourism," 1994.
6. Dobkin de Rios & Grob, "Hallucinogens, suggestibility," 1994.
7. Heelas, *New Age,* 1996.
8. Dobkin de Rios & Janiger, *LSD,* 2003; Masters & Houston, *Varieties,* 1966.
9. Berg, *Deconstructing,* 2003.
10. Dobkin de Rios, *Hallucinogens,* 1984.
11. Winkelman, "Drug tourism," 2005.
12. Lucas, "Not passing acid test," 2005.
13. Dobkin de Rios, *Visionary vine,* 1984.
14. Cushman, "Empty self," 1990.
15. Seguin, *Folklore psychiatry,* 1974.

Chapter 4 The New Shamans

1. Frecska, "Dangers," 2007.
2. Callaway et al., "Platelet," 1994.
3. Ibid.
4. Mabit, "Blending," 2002.
5. Siegel, *Intoxication,* 1989.
6. Dobkin de Rios & Grob, "Hallucinogens, suggestibility," 1994.

Chapter 5 The União do Vegetal and the U.S. Supreme Court

1. Baker, "Psychedelic sacraments," 2005; Wasson et al., "Road," 1998.
2. Durkheim, *Elementary,* 1951.

3. Dobkin de Rios et al., "Hallucinogens and redemption," 2002.
4. Dobkin de Rios & Grob, "Ayahuasca cross-cultural," 2006.
5. Groisman & Dobkin de Rios, "Ayahuasca, U.S. Supreme Court," 2007; Groisman, *Transplanting,* 1999.
6. Calabrese, "Supreme Court," 2001; Feeney, "Legal bases," 2007.
7. Ibid.
8. Feeney, "Legal bases," 2007.
9. Brannigin, "Court," 2006.
10. Groisman, *Transplanting,* 1999.
11. MacCrae, "Ritual," 1999.
12. Ibid.
13. Barbosa et al., "Altered states," 2005.
14. Groisman, *Transplanting,* 1999.

Chapter 6 Globalization and the Future of Ayahuasca

1. Friedman, *Lexus,* 2000.
2. Doblin, "Maps 20th anniversary," 2006.
3. Reko, *Magische,* 1949.
4. Moreno & Delgado, "Psilocybin," 2007.
5. Feeney, "Legal bases," 2007.
6. Adelaars, "Psychedelic rituals," 1997.
7. Tupper, "Globalization," 2006.
8. Tupper, *Ayahuasca healing,* n.d.; York, "New Age," 2001.
9. Ibid.
10. Dobkin de Rios, *Hallucinogens,* 1984.
11. Dobkin de Rios & Smith, "Function of drug," 1977.
12. Tupper, "Globalization," 2006; Tupper, *Ayahuasca healing,* n.d.
13. Grob et al., "Human psychopharmacology," 1994.
14. Winkelman, *Shamanism,* 2000.
15. Montagne, "Psychedelic," 2007.
16. Bronfman, personal communication, October 2007.

GLOSSARY

Alto Mesayoc Andean shaman with high level of knowledge

Ayahuasca A woody vine from South America with hallucinogenic properties

Ayahuascamama Mother spirit of the ayahuasca vine

Banco Term for mestizo ayahuasca healer with high level of knowledge

Banisteriopsis Botanical name for ayahuasca

Bomanuna Shipibo indigenous shamans who can transport themselves to other planes and who enter special states of consciousness, for example, seeing vidente phenomena

Brujería Witchcraft

Brujo Witch or evildoer who takes money or goods to harm or kill an individual's enemy

Bufeo Sweet-water dolphin

Burracheira Portuguese word for altered state induced by ayahuasca ingestion

Chacapa Plant leaves bound together to create a drumming sound, used by ayahuasca healers during ceremonies

Chacruna Additive to ayahuasca, *Psychotropia viridis,* contains a Schedule 1 drug, dimethyltryptamine (DMT)

Chiricsanango Powerful hallucinogen used in witchcraft

Cocama-Cocamilla Tribal group descended from Tupi Guarani Indians of the Amazon basin

Curandero Spanish term for traditional healer

Dieta Special diets traditionally used by ayahuasca healers and required of clients prior to ingesting the ayahuasca tea

Iboga Psychedelic plant used in West Africa in Bwiti initiation ceremonies

Icaro Healing song sung during ayahuasca sessions to invoke spirit forces for healing

Mal Aire Negative energy of people

Mariri Healing songs sung during ayahuasca sessions, also called Icaros

Meraya Shipibo Indian shaman with deep knowledge of administration of medicinal plants and magic, "who sees things"

Mestizo Individual with native American and European biological mixture, who participates in Western culture

Mestre Religious elder in the UDV Church in Brazil

Preparo Ceremony in the UDV Church to prepare large amounts of ayahuasca tea for ritual use

Pusanga Term for love magic potions

Rao Yoshin Intrinsic spirit of a plant or animal that shamans or brujos can take over in order to use its power to heal or harm

Saladera Misfortune illness believed caused by witchcraft and placing of salt over a person's threshold

San Pedro A mescaline cactus used in folk healing in the Peruvian coast; included in some neo-shamans' activities

Santo Daime Brazilian new religion that utilizes ayahuasca as a sacrament

Shiripiari Shaman among the Ashaninka Indians with high level of knowledge

Spiritualists Religious groups throughout Latin America who believe in communication with other realms and spirits of the dead

Takiwasi A healing center in Tarapoto, Peru that utilizes ayahuasca shamanism and Roman Catholic ritual in treating drug addicts and alcoholics; directed by a French psychiatrist, Jacques Mabit

Toé Powerful hallucinogen used in witchcraft

União do Vegetal (UDV) Brazilian religion that utilizes ayahuasca as a sacrament in church rituals

Vegetalista A plant doctor

Vidente Seer, an individual believed capable of seeing into the future

Virote Witchcraft dart believed by indigenous peoples of the Amazon to be introduced into enemy's body to cause illness and death

REFERENCES

Adelaars, A. (1997). Psychedelic rituals in the Netherlands. In C. Ratsch & J. Baker (Eds.), *Yearbook for ethnomedicine and the study of consciousness, 6–78*. Berlin, Germany: Verlag fur Wissenschaft und Bildung.

Baker, J. (2005). Psychedelic sacraments. *Journal of Psychoactive Drugs, 37*(2), 179–188.

Barbosa, P.C., Giglio, J.S., Dalgalarrondo, P. (2005). Altered states of consciousness and short term psychological after-effects induced by first-time ritual use of ayahuasca in an urban center in Brazil. *Journal of Psychoactive Drugs, 37*(2), 193–202.

Berg, A.A. (2003). *Deconstructing travel: Cultural perspectives on tourism.* Walnut Creek, CA: Altamira Press.

Bianchi, A., & Samorini, G. (1997). Plants in association with ayahuasca. In C. Ratsch & J. Baker (Eds.), *Yearbook for ethnomedicine and the study of consciousness.* Berlin, Germany: Verlag fur Wissenschaft und Bildung.

Brannigin, W. (2006). Court allows for use of hallucinogenic tea. Retrieved February 21, 2008, from http://www.maps.org/sys/nq.pl?id=787&fmt=page.

Bruner, E.M. (2006). *Culture on tour: Ethnographies of travel.* Chicago: University of Chicago Press.

Calabrese, J.D. (2001). The Supreme Court versus peyote: Consciousness alteration, cultural psychiatry and the dilemma of contemporary subcultures. *Anthropology of Consciousness, 12*(2), 4–19.

Callaway, J.C., Airaksinen, M.M., McKenna, D., Glacus, B., & Grob, C. (1994). Platelet serotonin uptake sites increased in drinkers of ayahuasca. *Psychopharmacology, 116,* 385–387.

Catholic Encyclopedia. (2003). Volume V11. Online edition. John Cardinal Farley. Archbishop of New York. Retrieved October 27, 2006, from http://www.newadvent.org.

Coppens, W., & David-Cato, J. (1971). El yopo entre los Cuiva-Guahibo: Aspectos etnográficos y farmacológicos. *Antropológica, 28,* 3–24.

Cushman, P. (1990). Why the self is empty: Toward a historically situated psychology. *American Psychology, 45*(5), 599–611.

Dobkin de Rios, M. (1969). Curanderismo psicodélico en el Peru. Continuidad y cambio. Mesa redonda de ciencias prehistóricas y antropológicas. Lima: Catholic University of Peru.

Dobkin de Rios, M. (1969). Fortune's malice: Divination, psychotherapy and folk medicine in Peru. *Journal of American Folklore, 82*(324), 132–141.

Dobkin de Rios, M. (1974). The influence of psychotropic flora and fauna on Maya religion. *Current Anthropology, 154*(2), 147–165.

Dobkin de Rios, M. (1981). Saladera—A culture-bound misfortune syndrome in the Peruvian Amazon. *Culture, Medicine and Psychiatry, 5,* 193–213.

Dobkin de Rios, M. (1984). *Hallucinogens: Cross-cultural perspective.* Prospect Hts., IL: Waveland Press.

Dobkin de Rios, M. (1984). The *vidente* phenomenon in third world traditional healing: An Amazonian example. *Medical Anthropology, 8,*(1), 60–70.

Dobkin de Rios, M. (1984). *Visionary vine: Hallucinogenic healing in the Peruvian Amazon.* Prospect Hts., IL: Waveland Press.

Dobkin de Rios, M. (1989). Plant hallucinogens and power in the pre-Colombian art of ancient Peru. In C. Ward (Ed.), *Altered states of consciousness and mental health.* New York: Sage Publishing.

Dobkin de Rios, M. (1992). *Amazon healer: The life and times of an urban shaman.* Bridport, England: Prism Press.

Dobkin de Rios, M. (1992). Twenty-five years of hallucinogenic studies in cross-cultural perspective. Newsletter, *Society for the Anthropology of Consciousness, 4*(1), 1–8.

Dobkin de Rios, M. (1994). Drug tourism in the Amazon. Newsletter, *Society for the Anthropology of Consciousness, 5*(1), 16–19. American Anthropological Association.

Dobkin de Rios, M. (1999). Shamanism and ontology: An evolutionary perspective. In A. Schenk & C. Ratsch (Eds.), *What is a Shaman?* Berlin, Germany: Verlag fur Wissenschaft und Bilden.

Dobkin de Rios, M., & Grob, C. S. (1994). Hallucinogens, suggestibility and adolescence in cross-cultural perspective. In C. Ratsch & J. Baker (Eds.), *Yearbook for ethnomedicine and the study of consciousness, 3,* 113–132. Berlin, Germany: Verlag fur Wissenschaft und Bildung.

Dobkin de Rios, M., & Grob, C. S. (2006). Ayahuasca use in cross-cultural perspective. *Journal of Psychoactive Drugs, 37*(2), June (theme issue).

Dobkin de Rios, M., & Grob, C. S. (2006). Interview with Jeffrey Bronfman, Representative Mestre for the União do Vegetal Church in the United States. *Journal of Psychoactive Drugs, 37*(2), 189–192.

Dobkin de Rios, M., Grob, C. S., & Baker, J. R. (2002). Hallucinogens and redemption. *Journal of Psychoactive Drugs, 34*(3), 239–248.

Dobkin de Rios, M., & Janiger, O. (2003). *LSD, spirituality and the creative process.* Rochester, VT: Inner Traditions.

Dobkin de Rios, M., & Rumrrill, R. (2005). Interview with Guillermo Arrévalo, a Shipibo urban Shaman, by Roger Rumrrill. *Journal of Psychoactive Drugs, 37*(2), 203–208.

Dobkin de Rios, M., & Smith, D. E. (1977). The function of drug rituals in human society: Continuities and changes. *Journal of Psychoactive Drugs, 9*(3), 269–276.

Doblin, R. (2006). *MAPS 20th Anniversary Financial Report, xvi*(30), 2–12.

Durkheim, E. (1951). *The elementary forms of the religious life.* New York: Collier Books. (Original work published 1932)

Eysenck, H.J. (1975). *Encyclopedia of psychology: Vol. 2.* (pp. 1–12). Bungay. New Guinea.

Feeney, K. (2007). The legal bases for religious peyote use. In M.J. Winkelman & T.B. Roberts (Eds.), *Psychedelic medicine* (pp. 233–250). Westport, CT: Praeger.

Frecska, E. (2007). Dangers and contraindications in therapeutic applications of hallucinogens. In M.J. Winkelman & T.B. Roberts (Eds.), *Psychedelic medicine* (pp. 69–96). Westport, CT: Praeger.

Freud, S. (1989). *The future of an illusion.* S. James, Ed. New York: Doubleday.

Friedman, T.L. (2000). *The Lexus and the olive tree.* New York: Anchor Books.

Gehricke, J.G., et al. (2007). Smoking to self-medicate attentional and emotional dysfunctions. *Nicotine & Tobacco Research, 9,* 523–536.

Grob, C.S. (2007). The use of psilocybin in patients with advanced cancer and existential anxiety. In M.J. Winkelman & T.B. Roberts (Eds.), *Psychedelic medicine* (pp. 205–216). Westport, CT: Praeger.

Grob, C.S. & Dobkin de Rios, M. (1992). Adolescent drug use in cross-cultural perspective. *Journal of Drug Issues, 22*(1), 121–138.

Grob, C.S., McKenna, D., Callaway, J., Brito, G.S., Neves, G., & Oberlander, O. (1994.) Human psychopharmacology of hoasca, a plant hallucinogen used in ritual context in Brazil. *Journal of Nervous and Mental Disease, 184*(2), 86–94.

Groisman, A. (1999). *Transplanting contexts: Cultural frontiers and transcultural knowledge in the expansion of ayahuasca cults to Europe.* Unpublished manuscript.

Groisman, A., & Dobkin de Rios, M. (2007). Ayahuasca, the U.S. Supreme Court, and the UDV-U.S. government case: Culture, religion, and implications of a legal dispute. In M.J. Winkelman & T.B. Roberts (Eds.), *Psychedelic medicine.* Westport, CT: Praeger.

Halpern, J.H., & Pope, H.G. (2001). Hallucinogens on the Internet: A vast new source of underground drug information. *American Journal of Psychiatry, 158*(3), 481–483.

Heelas, P. (1996). *The New Age movement. The celebration of the self and The sacralization of modernity.* London: Blackwell.

Krippner, S. (1999). Close encounters of the shamanic kind: From meetings to models. In A. Schenk & C. Ratsch (Eds.), *What is a shaman?* Berlin, Germany: Verlag fur Wissenschaft und Bildung.

Lathrap, D. (1979). *The upper Amazon.* New York: Thames and Hudson.

Lucas, M. (2005). On not passing the acid test: Bad trips and initiation. *Anthropology of Consciousness, 16*(1), 25–27.

Luna, E. (1984). The concept of plants as teachers among four mestizo shamans of Iquitos, northeastern Peru. *Journal of Ethnopharmacology, 111*(2), 135–156.

Mabit, J. (2002). Blending traditions: Using indigenous medicinal knowledge to treat drug addiction. *MAPS Bulletin, 12*(2), 25–32.

Mabit, J., & Sieber, C. (2006). The evolution of a pilot program utilizing ayahuasca in the treatment of drug addictions. *Shaman's Drum*.

MacCrae, E. (1999). The ritual and religious use of ayahuasca in contemporary Brazil. *DPF XII Policy Manual* (pp. 47–50). W. Taylor, W. Stewart, R. Hopkins, & K. Ehlers, Eds. Washington DC: The Drug Policy Foundation.

Masters, R., & Houston, J. (1966). *The varieties of psychedelic experience*. New York: Delta Publishing.

Montagne, M. (2007). Psychedelic therapy for treatment of depression. In M.J. Winkelman & T.B. Roberts (Eds.), *Psychedelic medicine*. Westport, CT: Praeger.

Moreno, F., & Delgado, P.L. (2007). Psilocybin treatment of obsessive compulsive disorder. In M.J. Winkelman & T.B. Roberts (Eds.), *Psychedelic medicine*. Westport, CT: Praeger.

Ortega y Gasset, J. (1992). *The revolt of the masses*. New York: W.W. Norton & Co. (Original work published 1932)

Owen-Kostelnik, J., Reppucci, N., & Meyer, J.R. (2006). Testimony and interrogation of minors. *American Psychologist, 61*(4), 286–304.

Reko, V.A. (1949). *Magische gifte: rausch-und betaubungsmittle der neuen welt* (pp. 65–76). Stuttgart, Germany: Ferdinand Enke Verlag.

Riba, J., et al. (2004). Effects of South American psychoactive beverage ayahuasca on regional brain electrical activity in humans: A functional neuro-imaging study using low-resolution electromagnetic tomography. *Neuropsychology, 50*, 89–101.

Rivier, L., & Lindgren, J. (1972). Ayahuasca, the South American hallucinogenic drink: An ethno-botanical and chemical investigation. *Journal of Economic Botany, 23*(1), 101–29.

Rodd, R. (2006). Piaroa sorcery and the navigation of negative affect: To be aware, to turn away. *Anthropology of Consciousness, 17*(1), 35–64.

Santo Daime. (2007). Alternative religions' profiles. Retrieved September 21, 2007, from http://www.santodaime.org.

Seguin, C.A. (1974). *Folklore psychiatry*. Lima, Peru: Ediciones Edmar.

Seligman, M. (2002). *Learned optimism: How to change your mind and your life*. New York: Free Press.

Siegel, R.K. (1989). *Intoxication: Life in pursuit of artificial paradise*. New York: Simon and Schuster.

Simon, H.A. (1990). A mechanism for social selection and successful altruism. *Science, 250*, 1665–1668.

Siskind, J. (1973). Visions and cures among the Sharanahua. In M.J. Harner (Ed.), *Hallucinogens and shamanism* (pp. 28–39). New York: Oxford University Press.

Sjoberg, B.M., & Hollister, E. (1965). The effects of psychotomimetic drugs on primary suggestibility. *Psychopharmacologia* (Berlin), *8*, 251–262.

Skinner, B.F. (1971). *Beyond freedom and dignity*. New York: A. Knopf.

Sklerov J.B., Levine, K., More, A., King, T., & Fowler, D. (2005). A fatal intoxication following the ingestion of 5-methoxy-N, N-dimethyltryptamine in an ayahuasca preparation. *Journal of Analytical Toxicology, 29*, 838–841.

Smith, H. (2005). Do drugs have religious import? A forty year follow-up. In R. Walsh & C. S. Grob (Eds.), *Higher wisdom: Eminent elders explore the continuing impact of psychedelics*. Albany, NY: State University of New York Press.

Stephens, R. S. (1999). Cannabis and hallucinogens. In B. S. McCrady & E. E. Epstein (Eds.), *Addictions: A comprehensive guidebook* (pp. 121–140). New York: Oxford University Press.

Tart, C. S. (1969). *Altered state of consciousness*. New York: John Wiley and Sons.

Tournon, J. (2002). La merma magica. Vida e historia de los Shipibo-Conibo del Ucayali. Lima, Peru: CAAAP (Centro Amazonico de Antropologia y Aplicacion Practica).

Tupper, K. W. (2006). The globalization of ayahuasca: Harm reduction or benefit maximization? *International Journal of Drug Policy*.

Tupper, K. W. (n.d.). *Ayahuasca healing beyond the Amazon: The globalization of a traditional indigenous entheogenic practice*. Unpublished manuscript.

União do Vegetal [UDV]. (2007). Retrieved March 6, 2007, from http://www.udv.org.br/ and http://www.udvusa.com/.

Wasson, R. G., et al. (1998). *The road to Eleusis: Unveiling the secret of the mysteries*. Los Angeles, CA: Hermes Press.

Winkelman, M. (2000). *Shamanism: The neural ecology of consciousness and healing*. Westport, CT: Bergin and Garvey.

Winkelman, M. (2005). Drug tourism or spiritual healing? Ayahuasca seekers in Amazonia. *Journal of Psychoactive Drugs, 37*(2), 209–218.

York, M. (2001). New Age commodification and appropriation of spirituality. *Journal of Contemporary Religion, 16*(3), 361–372.

INDEX

ABOUT THE AUTHORS

Marlene Dobkin de Rios is a medical anthropologist who has conducted fieldwork in the Peruvian Amazon and the coast on plant hallucinogens and healing. She is an associate clinical professor of psychiatry and human behavior at the University of California–Irvine and is professor emerita of anthropology at California State University–Fullerton. De Rios has spearheaded research on the plant hallucinogen ayahuasca in Peru, Brazil, and the United States. The author of six books and several hundred articles on hallucinogens and culture, she resides in southern California.

Roger Rumrrill is a well-known Peruvian journalist and the author of 25 books. He is a recognized expert on Amazon themes, including narco-trafficking, biological wealth of the Amazon, and social and cultural issues of indigenous peoples in Peru and other regions of Latin America.